CORE STRENGTH FOR 50+

A Customized Program for Safely Toning Ab, Back & Oblique Muscles

Dr. Karl Knopf

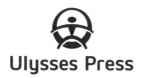

Ulysses Press

Published in the United States by
Ulysses Press
P.O. Box 3440
Berkeley, CA 94703
www.ulyssespress.com

ISBN: 978-1-61243-101-7
Library of Congress Control Number 2012940419

Printed in Canada by Marquis Book Printing

10 9 8 7 6 5 4

Acquisitions: Kelly Reed
Managing editor: Claire Chun
Editor: Lily Chou
Proofreader: Lauren Harrison
Indexer: Sayre Van Young
Production: Judith Metzener
Cover design: what!design @ whatweb.com
Cover photographs: front © Joshua Hodge Photography/istockphoto.com;
    back © Rapt Productions
Interior photographs: © Rapt Productions except page 12 muscle illustration
    © Sebastian Kaulitzki/shutterstock.com, page 17 skeleton © leonello calvetti/
    shutterstock.com
Models: Karl Knopf, Toni Silver, Jeff Rankin

Distributed by Publishers Group West

Please Note
This book has been written and published strictly for informational purposes,
and in no way should be used as a substitute for actual instruction with quali-
fied professionals. The author and publisher are providing you with information
in this work so that you can have the knowledge and can choose, at your own
risk, to act on that knowledge. The author and publisher also urge all readers to
be aware of their health status and to consult health care professionals before
beginning any health program.

CORE
STRENGTH
FOR 50+

contents

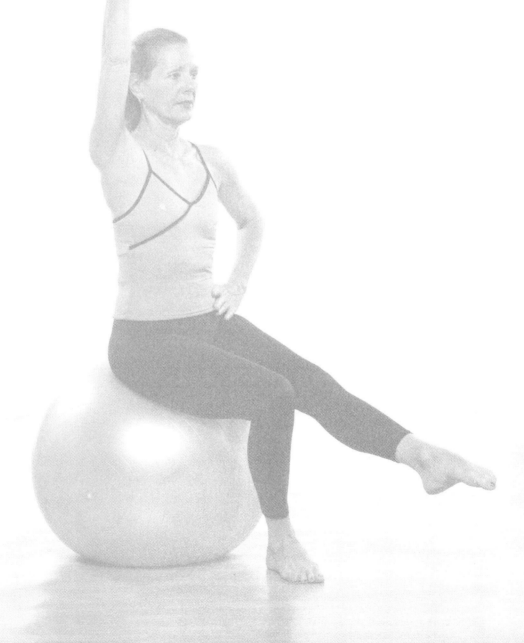

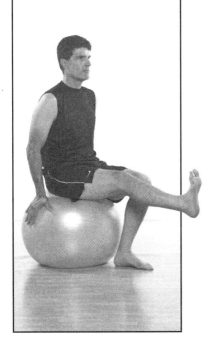

introduction

The "core" is the powerhouse of the body. When the concept of "core strength" training was first introduced, the core was considered to be only the abdominal region and the low back area. Nowadays, some experts consider the core to be the region from the tops of the legs to the shoulder area. With its roots in back rehabilitation, core training was later thought to be useful in sports performance. Today, core training needs to be a part of every-day exercise programs.

Having an aligned and strong yet flexible core can take the load off the vertebral column and discs, which results in improved function and less discomfort and pain. It'll also assist you in activities of daily living, help improve posture, and maybe even boost appearance and foster athletic performance.

Consider a tower of blocks: If the blocks aren't lined up properly and a load is placed on top of it, the middle portion often buckles and collapses. This is also what happens when we don't have a solid core. Some experts maintain that true core strength is the interaction of the total body. It's about improving functional fitness and reducing the strain on the spinal region. Core strength-ening goes far beyond just having a flat stomach and six-pack abs.

Core Strength for 50+ is very different from other core train-ing books because it focuses on providing comprehensive, total-body core-strengthening options. The exercises described in this book are based on the most recent scientific knowledge of how the spine responds to cor-rective exercise. Any exercise that doesn't have superior benefits and minimal risks was not included. Additionally, some traditional core exercises were transformed a bit to accommodate balance and joint issues often seen in the 50-plus person. By using *Core Strength for 50+*, you're well on your way to enhancing your spine's stability and re-educating correct muscle activation patterns.

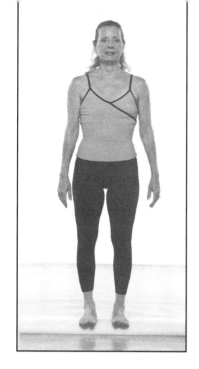

what is core strength?

Fitness fads come and go but core-strength training is not a passing trend. "Core strength" is *not* achieved by just doing a bunch of sit-ups; in addition, using heavy resistance is counterproductive. Rather, core strength is an integrated approach of systematic conditioning and correcting of muscular imbalances.

Too often people exercise their abdominals (or "abs") for aesthetic reasons, but correct core strength is gained through proper activation of specific muscles in a coordinated fashion. Proper core training teaches you to engage and protect your back even when you're not even thinking about your core. You'll know you mastered core training if you automatically engage your core muscles when you open a door, swing a golf club, get up from sitting, or lift something.

The roots of core training stem from sound back rehabilitation. The average fitness follower or anyone who has ever had a bad back is familiar with the terms "core stability" and "core train-

ing." Core training is also known as "dynamic lumbar stabilization."

Core training became very common in the early 1980s and received the most acclaim when used by San Francisco 49er quarterback Joe Montana. The belief was that stabilization of the lumbar region would guard your low back by using your own body to build your own lumbar support. Patients were taught how to find the most balanced, pain-free position while in a static position and then progress to being able to locate that position in a variety of dynamic movements. This approach was so successful with clients who had intervertebral disc problems as well as facet joint involvement and other

muscular imbalance issues that it was incorporated into fitness and sports conditioning routines for the young and old.

Core Strength vs. Core Stabilization

Core training goes by many names, such as core stabilization and core strengthening, to name the most common ones. They all generally agree that the abdominal and low back muscles must have the right amount of strength, endurance, and flexibility, as well as the muscle memory of knowing automatically when and how to engage and relax the core set of muscles. However, people often overlook the muscular balance that's required for a strong core, and only do sit-ups and back extensions without addressing all the subtle changes of posture and deep-lying muscles. This may lead to physical problems down the line.

When strengthening your core, be sure to train both the superficial and deep-lying muscles in the front, back, and sides of the body. Your body needs a combination of muscular endurance to handle prolonged sitting and standing, and enough strength in that region to keep your posture long and tall.

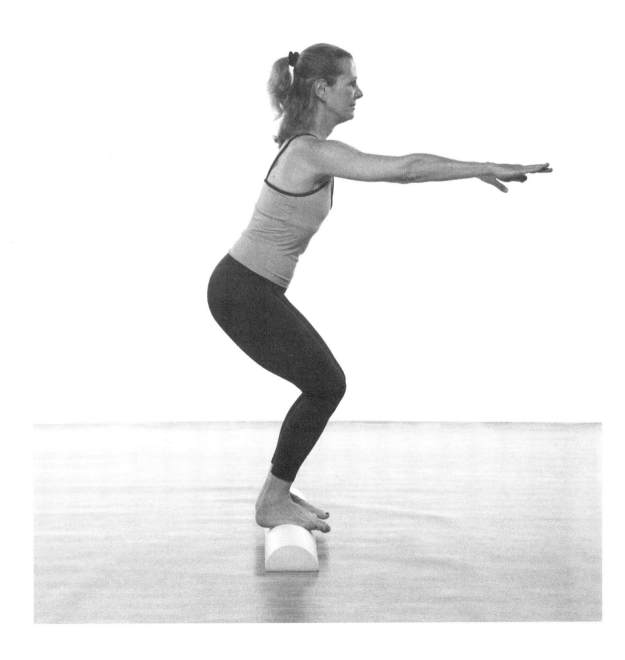

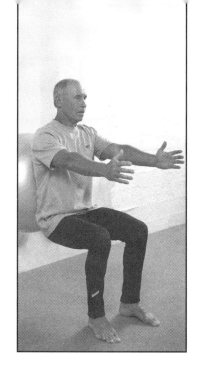

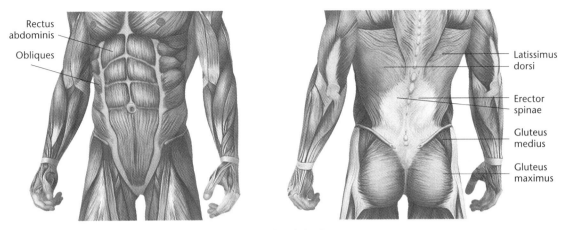

where is the core?

The "core" of anything is the central foundation of the structure, whether it's the core of an apple or the core of a nuclear reactor. Although no one universal definition of "core" exists, most people refer to the abdominal wall muscles in the front of the body and the muscles of the back that run up and down the spine as the core of the human body. Sometimes the gluteal region gets included.

The core is a complicated arrangement of bones, nerves, ligaments, tendons, and supporting muscle configurations. Understanding the locations and roles of the muscles that comprise the core will motivate you to keep participating in a core-strengthening routine day in and day out.

The core team is made up of a pole (the vertebral column) and guide wires (the muscles), and each member of your core team has a specific role. The core muscle group includes the transverse abdominis, internal and external obliques, rectus abdominis, and erector spinae.

The *transverse abdominis* is the deepest-lying layer of fibers of the abdominal wall. The transverse abdominis provides compression to the internal organs and serves as nature's back brace. Some physical therapists believe that the transverse abdominis is the most important element of core training.

The *internal and external obliques* are the muscles on the sides of the body. They're engaged when you twist to reach and grab something.

The *rectus abdominis* is the muscle that flexes the vertebral column. We're most familiar with this muscle because it gives us the six pack. It also helps stabilize the pelvis when walking.

The *erector spinae* group is responsible for extending the back. It's made up of three distinct muscles: the iliocostalis, the longissimus, and the spinalis. The erectors add stability to the trunk area and are also the primary muscles that help us stand erect.

Rectus abdominis
Obliques
Latissimus dorsi
Erector spinae
Gluteus medius
Gluteus maximus

Major Muscles of the Core

When the core muscles are properly trained, they lead to improved posture and back protection.

Current research also suggests that the diaphragm assists spinal stability via a hydraulic consequence on the abdominal hollow space by increasing intra-abdominal pressure, often seen in weightlifters who bear down when doing a heavy lift. For years the transverse abdominis was considered the key component for spinal stabilization training. However, today it's understood that the "deep core" muscles and the diaphragm need to work in a coordinated manner to provide an ideal platform from which the more superficial muscles can operate.

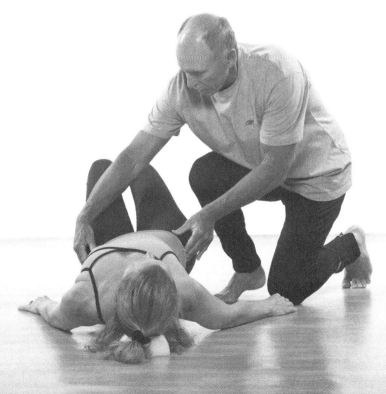

Author Karl Knopf makes some adjustments.

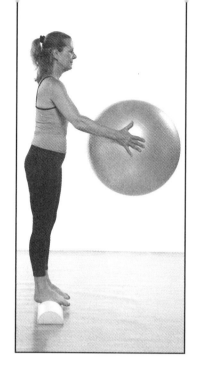

benefits of a strong core

Much like replacing the plumbing under your house, core strengthening is often not visible. No one will ever see what you've done but if it's not working, things can really become a mess. Being fit doesn't necessarily translate into being highly aware of your core muscles. Oftentimes, a fit, athletic person can more easily substitute other muscles to perform the functions associated with the core.

The benefits of having a strong core include improved posture, which allows you to present a more youthful appearance, and balance. It also means less load on the lumbar region of your low back, reducing the risk of injury to any arthritic joints and discs in addition to pain. Performance in sports and recreational pursuits is also boosted.

Core Strength and Back Pain Prevention

Having a solid core is analogous to the concept of keeping a radio tower upright. A radio tower is installed with guide wires to keep the tower straight and tall. If one set of wires is lax and another set is too tight, the tower becomes misaligned. The same applies to the back, with the spine being the radio tower and the muscles of the body being the guide wires. If one set of muscles is too tight from overuse and the others too lax from lack of use, the spine becomes unstable and is at high risk for injury. Muscle imbalances, along with poor body mechanics and age, are believed to be a factor in low back issues.

It's important to keep in mind that "back pain" is a very generic term and can range in severity from simple overexertion to a herniated disc to something very serious (e.g., pain referred from a major organ). That's why a medical doctor should evaluate persistent, unrelenting low back pain.

That said, certain kinds of back pain can be prevented or reversed by proper core strengthening. A comprehensive core-strength training program can be thought of as building your own back brace to protect your spine, along with learning proper biomechanics and maintaining flexibility to avoid muscle spasms.

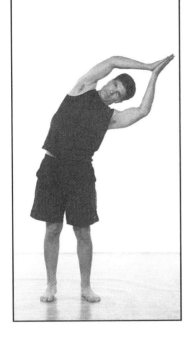

core training the right way

Core strengthening is all about improving functional fitness and reducing the strain on the spinal region. A well-designed core-strength program requires a delicate balance of core strength, core muscle endurance, proper body mechanics, and flexibility of the surrounding muscles (such as the hamstrings, quadriceps, iliopsoas, and the iliotibial band) that often contribute to low back imbalances.

Complete core-strength training requires a balanced multi-planar approach that includes a combination of isometric and dynamic exercises. While many of the exercises in this book look simple, it's critical that you master the subtleties of the movements through concentration and practice them until they become automatic before moving on to the next level.

Proper core stabilization has four basic stages:

Stage 1   Learn to contract deep-lying muscles.

Stage 2   Focus on endurance of the deep-lying muscles.

Stage 3   Challenge the core with arm movements once stabilization can be maintained.

Stage 4   Continue challenging the core.

The beauty of a core strength program is that it can be used as both a preventative and rehabilitative back-care wellness tool. The desired outcomes of a good core-strength program are:

• A solid core that will protect the low back, reduce back injuries, and foster better low-back health

• Improved sports performance

• A better interdependence between the muscles on the front of the body and the back of the body, which will reduce fatigue and improve posture

To achieve these aspects, you can progress to performing the exercises in a supported position, such as supine, prone, kneeling, and standing, before finally incorporating dynamic movement. To truly improve core strength, meticulous body awareness is needed. Talking or listening to music while doing these exercises can detract from learning core stabilization, so no distractions are recommended. Core training requires total mind-body interaction. Just pounding out sit-ups to the latest tunes is not what core-strength training is all about.

10 Core-Training Tips

Here are 10 tips that will help you make the most of your core-training workout.

1. Core training can and should be done daily. If you're pressed for time, exercise the front side of your body one day and then exercise the posterior side of your body the next day.

2. Concentration and practice and then more concentration and more practice are the axiom of core training.

3. Train, don't make pain. Follow the two-hour rule: If you hurt more than two hours post-exercise, re-evaluate your exercise program and back off.

4. Better results occur when you cross-train—in addition to core training, include a regular walking program with comfortable shoes or participate in a water-exercise program.

5. Avoid doing core exercises first thing in the morning. It's believed that intervertebral fluid pressure in the spinal region is higher in the morning and can cause problems.

6. Focus on core muscle endurance rather than aiming to make the muscles overly strong.

7. Sad but true, there's no ideal set of exercises for everyone. Your exercises need to evolve and adapt according to your functional goals and pain issues. Some people will do core exercises for rehabilitative purposes and others for general fitness and prevention, while others do it to enhance athletic performance. Therefore, use your inner wisdom when selecting and designing a core strength program.

8. Don't expect quick results. It'll take a long time to learn to perform the exercises correctly and mindfully. The goal of core training is instinctually knowing how to properly engage your core muscles while performing activities of daily living.

9. Practice braced breathing and learn diaphragmatic breathing (see page 35).

10. When performing static exercises, don't hold your breath. If you have any cardiovascular issues, avoid static exercises.

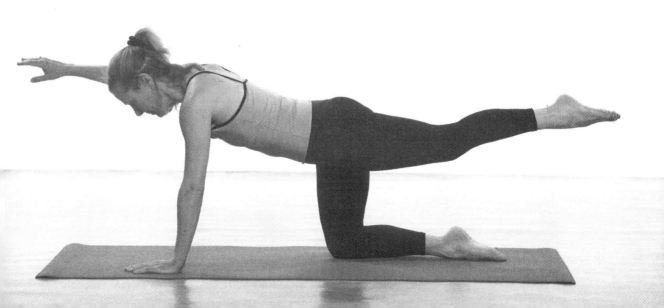

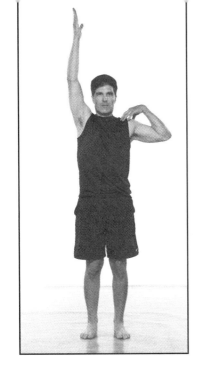

the importance of posture

I work with many 50-plus folks, and they're often concerned about their appearance. They'll spend great amounts of money on hair products, facials, and clothes but spend little or no time on their posture. To better understand posture's role in how we look, check out a local high school play and see how the actor portrays an old person—all hunched over!

If you want to look young, stand tall. If you want to look thinner, stand tall. Core training is all about improving how you look and feel. Every time I do my core-strengthening exercises, I think about how they'll help me stand straight and therefore improve my appearance.

As you can see from the illustration of the human spine on page 17, the neck (called the cervical spine) curves slightly forward. The middle portion of the spine (thoracic spine) is curved outward. The lower portion of the back (lumbar spine) curves inward, presenting a lordotic curve. Although the vertebral column has three natural curves, sometimes as a result of misuse, disuse, or abuse, these curves become overly exaggerated and can contribute to back problems.

A visual that might assist you to better understand the concept is to picture a brand-new tube of toothpaste and stand it on one end. When all the forces are exerting equal pressure, the tube stands up easily. Now squeeze the toothpaste a few times with some spots going in and other parts pushed out. Now try to stand it up. I doubt that it'll stay up.

Learning to sit, stand, and move in the most biomechanical manner is foundational. A properly aligned back has a gentle "S" curve. When it's in the safest position to avoid excessive forces to the spine and discs, it's called

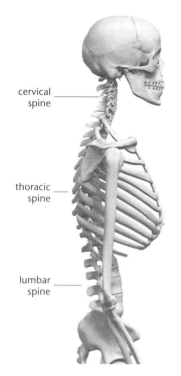

cervical spine

thoracic spine

lumbar spine

Human spine

neutral spine. Everyone has their own neutral spine position. This is how you find it while standing:

- Stand with your weight evenly distributed over both feet and your knees slightly bent.
- Using your abdominal muscles, tilt your hips slowly forward and back. Imagine you have a cup of water resting on your belly and are trying to tip water out of it. Find a position that feels most comfortable for you (ideally a balanced position from which the water in that cup would not spill). Movement occurs at the hip-

hinge joint. Once you locate it, lock in that position.

- Make sure your hips and shoulders are aligned and that the distance from your belly button to your sternum is far apart.
- After this adjustment, you may need to re-align the hip-hinge joint again.
- Align your ears over your shoulders, your shoulders over your hips, and your hips over your ankles.

The goal is to put this "feeling" into muscle memory so you can maintain the correct position throughout the day. While this is meant to be natural, it can take some time to get used to.

Another way to find neutral spine is to stand with your spine against a corner or wall and align the base of your skull, your mid-back and tailbone, allowing for the natural arches. Look

in a mirror or ask a friend: Are your ears over your shoulders, shoulders over your hips, and hips over your ankles?

In proper core training, learning proper pelvic positioning is pivotal. Let's review the various positions that the exercises in this book use. The ultimate goal is for you to be able to stand, run, and jump and always have your back in a self-protected position.

Lying Position

Whether you're lying on the floor or a roller, flatten and arch your back until you find a comfortable position. Your back shouldn't be completely flat on the ground.

Tabletop Position

While on your hands and knees, find neutral position, engage your abdominal muscles, and keep your spine stabilized. Ideally, a broom handle should be able to

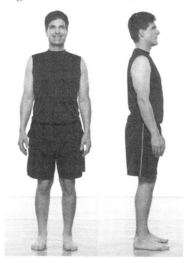

Neutral spine while standing

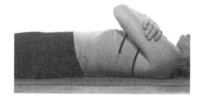

Neutral spine when lying down

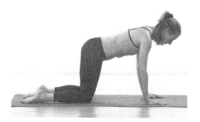

Tabletop position

As basic as the next statement will appear, it's critical that, when performing core-stabilization exercises, you understand how to lower and raise yourself to/from the floor in a biomechanically correct manner. Improperly getting up and down from/to the floor contributes to low back pain. *Remember to maintain control of your torso during every phase of the movement. Think of your shoulders, hips, and spine as one unit.*

1–2 From standing, bend your knees and place both hands on the floor to lower yourself into a tabletop position.

3 Lower one hip to the floor, sitting like a mermaid.

4 Then lower yourself down on that side.

5 Once you're on your side, roll like a log onto your back, keeping your torso in one unit. Use your hands to assist if necessary. Once on the floor, align your spine and neck, and bend your knees and place your feet flat on the floor.

To get up, perform the process in reverse.

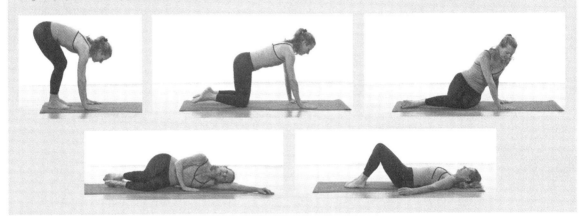

rest on your back from head to tailbone, with only a small arch in your low back area.

Sitting Position
Whether you're on a chair or ball, be sure to find neutral spine:
- Sit with both feet on the floor and both bones of your pelvis (not your tailbone) on the chair/ball.
- Your upper legs should be parallel with the floor, and your feet should be shoulder-width apart on the floor. Your weight is evenly distributed over all contact points.

- Your chest, shoulders, and head are up and out, with the maximum distance between your belly button and sternum.
- Avoid sitting with a rounded back and head forward; it could add stress to your discs.

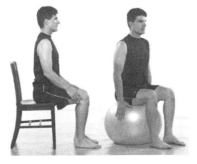

Sitting position

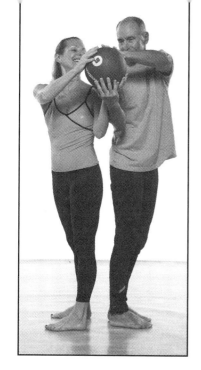

before you begin

Before embarking on a core-training program, first make sure that you're healthy enough to participate. If you have any existing health concerns, always consult with your health professional. Given that you're indeed healthy, make sure you're fit enough to get up and down from the floor. If not, please check out my book *Weights for 50+* to help you get stronger.

Core training is usually best done when the body is properly warmed up. Many people participate in this routine at the end of their exercise session or after a warm shower. Pay attention to your body and figure out the best times for it. The key is not to force your body to do things it's not ready for—train, don't strain.

To train safely, please keep these additional simple tips in mind:

• Listen to your body: If it hurts more two hours post-exercise than it did before you started, you did too much. Be smart and do less next time. Only YOU know your body best.

• If an exercise hurts, stop and reassess if that exercise is right for everyone. In addition, please note that not every exercise is right for everyone. What might be a perfect exercise for one person can contribute to further issues for another.

• If you experience numbness, please see a health care professional.

• Research has shown that unstable-surface training results in increased core muscle recruitment. However, do not progress to an unstable surface until you have the requisite balance skills. You can obtain adequate core conditioning without ever doing unstable-surface exercises. Always consider your safety first.

Equipment

Balance balls, foam rollers, and other tools can all be used to challenge the system, but they're not necessary to strengthen the core. In fact, if they're not used properly, they'll only contribute to muscle imbalances. Too often people rush to use a piece of equipment before they're ready. In core-strength training, perfect technique is vital.

The beauty of core training is that it requires no equipment. If you don't have the space for a ball, don't buy one. If you don't feel safe on a roller, don't use it. However, if you decide that you're ready for a new experience, here are some things to consider.

Stability Ball

When choosing a ball, make sure that when you sit on it, your upper legs and lower legs are at 90 degrees, and your shoulders are over your hips. The ball should also be safe for your body weight.

- The firmer the ball, the more challenging the exercise will be.
- Make sure that the floor surface is safe for both you and the ball—avoid sharp objects.
- Don't overestimate your ability—start with the basics.
- Have someone spot you if necessary.
- Only do those movements that are correct for your health status.

Foam Roller

A foam roller is a fun and challenging piece of equipment that can be purchased at most sporting goods stores, gyms, or physical therapy clinics. It has been reported to restore alignment, foster body awareness, and advance proper posture. Foam roller exercises can be done from numerous positions, including supine and kneeling.

The foam roller comes in various shapes, sizes, and densities. The selection of the correct roller depends on your height and body weight. The most common roller used for core-strength training is a full-length roller that's about three feet long. It comes in a semicircular or fully circular shape. Beginners do best with the semicircular shape, flat-side down; as they improve, they can flip the roller over. Once that becomes easy, a circular roller is a nice way to ramp up the challenge.

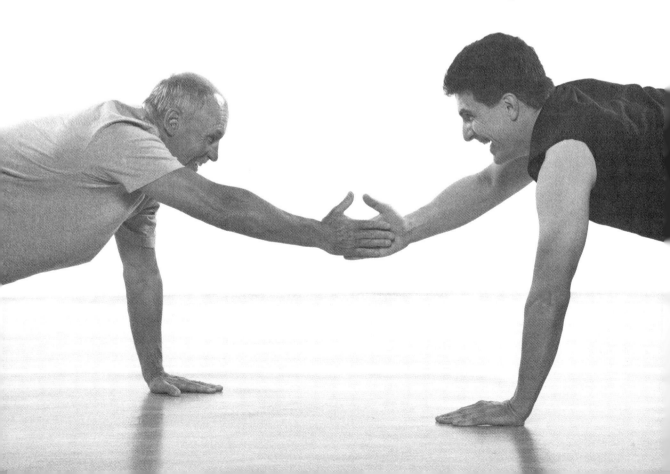

part 2

the

programs

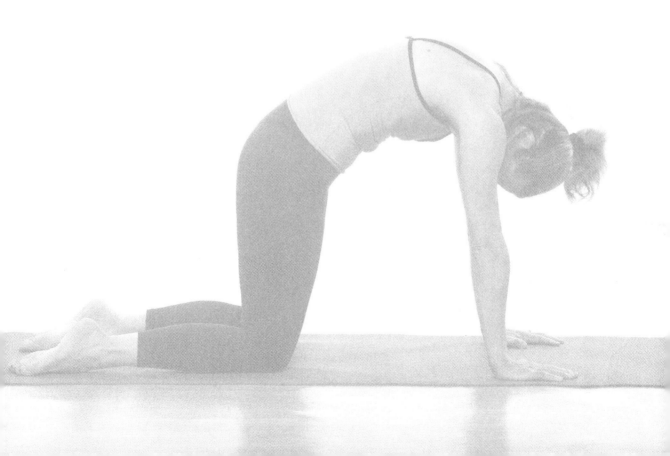

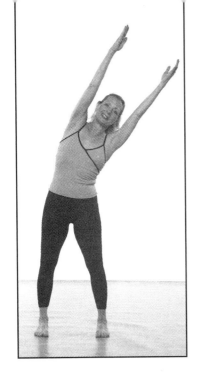

how to use this book

The key to a well-aligned core is to strengthen that which is weak and lengthen that which is inflexible. This section of *Core Strength for 50+* has eight different programs to help you improve your posture, prevent chronic low back issues, improve performance in recreational pursuits, and have a more youthful stature. Choose from equipment-free programs or those that use a variety of stability-building tools, or pick and choose from the exercises in Part 3 and create your own routine.

The programs have more exercises than you're expected to do. Focus on the particular aspects that are relevant to you, then select 5–6 exercises and do them for several weeks. Most people will be fine just doing a daily dose of levels 1 and/or 2. After that period, select another 5–6 exercises from the same level or the next. It's okay to select exercises from different levels as long as you're able to safely and properly perform them. This method keeps your routine more vibrant and prevents burnout. By inserting new exercises on a

regular basis, you also continue to challenge your core. When I teach classes, we never do the same core exercises every single time. Again, core training isn't like weight training, where each exercise works a specific muscle. Core training essentially works the entire core.

Keep in mind that you're encouraged to select those exercises that you enjoy or feel your body requires—this is *your* program. Some readers will need more back stabilization/strengthening exercises while others may need more mobility of the low back

and pelvic area. If you're having a particular concern, you may want to take this book to your health provider and ask them to select the exercises that meet your current health issue.

Every reader should start at the baseline of "beginner." Whether and how quickly you progress to the next level is determined by your particular competence at each level. The progression from one level to the next is very subjective and not at all like progression levels seen in weight training.

Unlike traditional strength training (which is all about numbers of reps), core-strength training blends the concepts of both strength training and endurance training (which focuses on how long can you perform a move before the muscular system fatigues). Perfect form and mindfulness are extremely important. If you can't perform a movement without maintaining stability, you're not performing the exercise correctly and are wasting your time. That said, when it comes to training the core, you can utilize a combination of both reps and/or duration:

Beginner: 10 reps or 30 sec
Intermediate: 15 reps or 45 sec
Advanced: 20 reps or 1 min
Super-Advanced: 30 sec or as many/as long as tolerated

These parameters are just suggestions. Determining whether you use duration or reps is a personal choice. It's always prudent to start with just a few and progress only as you feel confident to do so. As always, listen to your body and enjoy the process of strengthening your core.

The beauty of core-strength training is that it can be done anytime and anywhere with or without equipment. Some people perform core strengthening at the end of their exercise session. This can serve as a cool-down portion of their routine and is an ideal time to also stretch the muscles that influence core alignment. Regardless of when you do your core training, make sure to properly warm up your body for movement.

Everyone should start with the *supine floor exercises*, which focus on the muscles of the anterior side of the body. Master these moves before moving on to the *prone* (face-down), *tabletop* (hands-and-knees), and *plank* exercises. Once the tabletop and plank exercises become easier, you can challenge yourself some more by placing an unstable surface such as a pillow under your hands and/or knees or feet.

Safe positioning is paramount in performing the *foam roller exercises*. It'll take time to get used to maintaining proper alignment and stability on the roller. For this series, you may want to start with a half roller and place the flat side down. As you become more comfortable, flip the roller over and perform the movement with the rounded side down. Once you're proficient at that stage, try a full circular roller, and then progress to resting your feet on a pillow while doing the exercises to challenge yourself even more.

The major focus of the standing roller exercises is to encourage greater static and dynamic core stability. Since these moves require a good level of balance, you may want to place a chair alongside you or work next to a wall. Don't perform these moves if you're not 100 percent confident in your skill level. These are very advanced exercises and are not needed to obtain good core stability.

The *ball exercises* are a fun way to challenge yourself, but make sure you have adequate balance as well as space to perform the exercises. Doing exercises on an unstable surface is an excellent way to engage greater core muscular activation.

The *partner exercises* are for the extremely advanced person. Partner exercises require cooperation and communication between partners. It's not about competition. Partner training when done cooperatively can target specific muscle groups and functional movements. If you choose to do partner exercises, make sure you both understand the movement patterns of the drill and are willing to adjust to each other's level.

Remember: You don't need to do all of the exercises listed in each program during each session if you don't have time. However, if you do an exercise that addresses the muscles on the front of the body, try to follow it with an exercise that addresses the muscles on the back of the body. Additionally, if the program calls for ball or roller moves but you don't own either, it's fine to perform the equipment-free versions.

equipment-free program level 1

This level focuses on mastering the movements and toning your deeper-lying muscles. It'll meet the basic needs of anyone wishing to add a core-strengthening element to their existing fitness routine.

EQUIPMENT-FREE LEVEL 1

Warm up with some light aerobic exercise or a warm shower for at least 10 minutes before performing core training. Then select 5–6 exercises and do them for 10 reps or 30 seconds.

EXERCISE

Supine Foundational Position *p. 34*

Supine Leg Extension *p. 36*

Supine Arm Swing *p. 37*

Curl-Up *p. 43*

Pelvic Lift *p. 50*

Tabletop Arm Raise *p. 64*

Tabletop Leg Raise *p. 65*

Clam Shell *p. 63*

Mad Cat Stretch *p. 121*

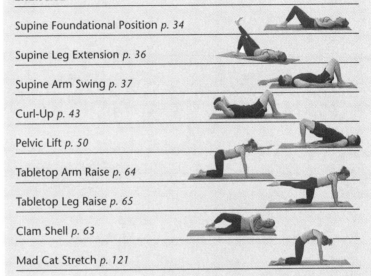

Remember to stretch after your workout. Select 3–5 exercises and hold for 30 seconds to 1 minute. See pages 105–21 for suggestions.

Level 2 introduces dynamic, compound exercises that progressively challenge the core.

EQUIPMENT-FREE LEVEL 2

Warm up with some light aerobic exercise or a warm shower for at least 10 minutes before performing core training. Then select 5–6 exercises and do them for 10 reps or 30 seconds.

EXERCISE

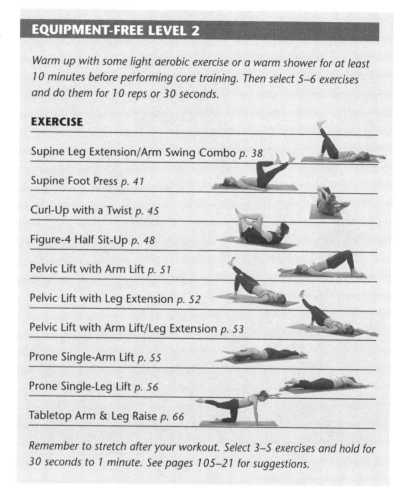

Supine Leg Extension/Arm Swing Combo *p. 38*

Supine Foot Press *p. 41*

Curl-Up with a Twist *p. 45*

Figure-4 Half Sit-Up *p. 48*

Pelvic Lift with Arm Lift *p. 51*

Pelvic Lift with Leg Extension *p. 52*

Pelvic Lift with Arm Lift/Leg Extension *p. 53*

Prone Single-Arm Lift *p. 55*

Prone Single-Leg Lift *p. 56*

Tabletop Arm & Leg Raise *p. 66*

Remember to stretch after your workout. Select 3–5 exercises and hold for 30 seconds to 1 minute. See pages 105–21 for suggestions.

equipment-free program level 3

This advanced program places a more rigorous demand on the core by introducing more complex elements. Most readers won't engage in all the exercises in this section. As with all the exercises in this book, form is critical and duration of how long you perform the movement is the goal.

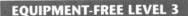

EQUIPMENT-FREE LEVEL 3

Warm up with some light aerobic exercise or a warm shower for at least 10 minutes before performing core training. Then select 5–6 exercises and do them for 10 reps or 30 seconds.

EXERCISE

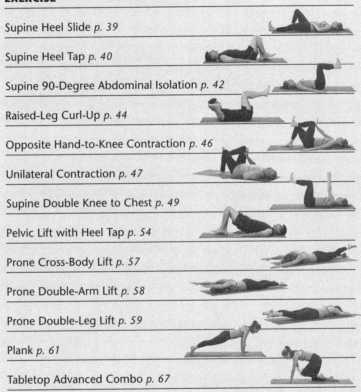

Supine Heel Slide *p. 39*

Supine Heel Tap *p. 40*

Supine 90-Degree Abdominal Isolation *p. 42*

Raised-Leg Curl-Up *p. 44*

Opposite Hand-to-Knee Contraction *p. 46*

Unilateral Contraction *p. 47*

Supine Double Knee to Chest *p. 49*

Pelvic Lift with Heel Tap *p. 54*

Prone Cross-Body Lift *p. 57*

Prone Double-Arm Lift *p. 58*

Prone Double-Leg Lift *p. 59*

Plank *p. 61*

Tabletop Advanced Combo *p. 67*

Remember to stretch after your workout. Select 3–5 exercises and hold for 30 seconds to 1 minute. See pages 105–21 for suggestions.

equipment-free program level 4

This super-advanced program is designed for the highly motivated. It's extremely challenging and also includes a fun partner move.

EQUIPMENT-FREE LEVEL 4

Warm up with some light aerobic exercise or a warm shower for at least 10 minutes before performing core training. Then select 5–6 exercises and do them for 10 reps or 30 seconds.

EXERCISE

Prone Double-Double *p. 60*

Side Plank *p. 62*

Plank to Side Salutation *p. 80*

Plank Clap *p. 104*

Remember to stretch after your workout. Select 3–5 exercises and hold for 30 seconds to 1 minute. See pages 105–21 for suggestions.

level 1

This level focuses on mastering the movements and toning your deeper-lying muscles. It'll meet the basic needs of anyone wishing to add a core-strengthening element to their existing fitness routine.

LEVEL 1

Warm up with some light aerobic exercise or a warm shower for at least 10 minutes before performing core training. Then select 5–6 exercises and do them for 10 reps or 30 seconds.

EXERCISE

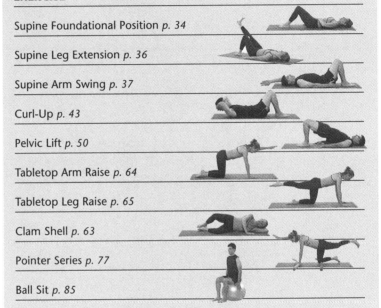

Supine Foundational Position *p. 34*

Supine Leg Extension *p. 36*

Supine Arm Swing *p. 37*

Curl-Up *p. 43*

Pelvic Lift *p. 50*

Tabletop Arm Raise *p. 64*

Tabletop Leg Raise *p. 65*

Clam Shell *p. 63*

Pointer Series *p. 77*

Ball Sit *p. 85*

Remember to stretch after your workout. Select 3–5 exercises and hold for 30 seconds to 1 minute. See pages 105–21 for suggestions.

level 2

This program introduces dynamic, compound exercises that progressively challenge the core. It also uses the foam roller, which you may choose to not use.

LEVEL 2

Warm up with some light aerobic exercise or a warm shower for at least 10 minutes before performing core training. Then select 5–6 exercises and do them for 10 reps or 30 seconds.

EXERCISE

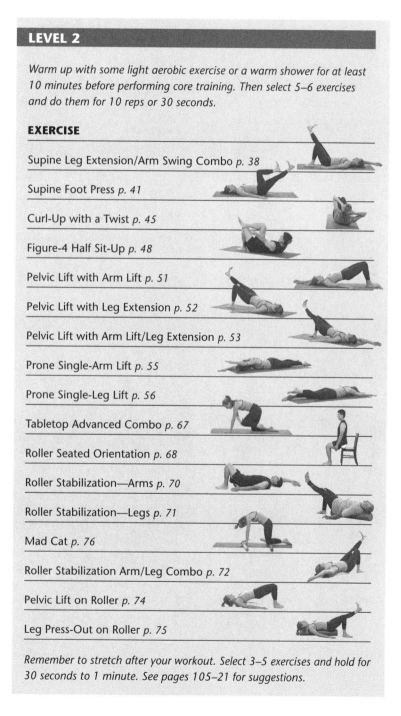

Supine Leg Extension/Arm Swing Combo *p. 38*

Supine Foot Press *p. 41*

Curl-Up with a Twist *p. 45*

Figure-4 Half Sit-Up *p. 48*

Pelvic Lift with Arm Lift *p. 51*

Pelvic Lift with Leg Extension *p. 52*

Pelvic Lift with Arm Lift/Leg Extension *p. 53*

Prone Single-Arm Lift *p. 55*

Prone Single-Leg Lift *p. 56*

Tabletop Advanced Combo *p. 67*

Roller Seated Orientation *p. 68*

Roller Stabilization—Arms *p. 70*

Roller Stabilization—Legs *p. 71*

Mad Cat *p. 76*

Roller Stabilization Arm/Leg Combo *p. 72*

Pelvic Lift on Roller *p. 74*

Leg Press-Out on Roller *p. 75*

Remember to stretch after your workout. Select 3–5 exercises and hold for 30 seconds to 1 minute. See pages 105–21 for suggestions.

level 3

This advanced program places a more rigorous demand on the core by introducing more complex elements. Most readers won't engage in all the exercises in this section. As with all the exercises in this book, form is critical and duration of how long you perform the movement is the goal.

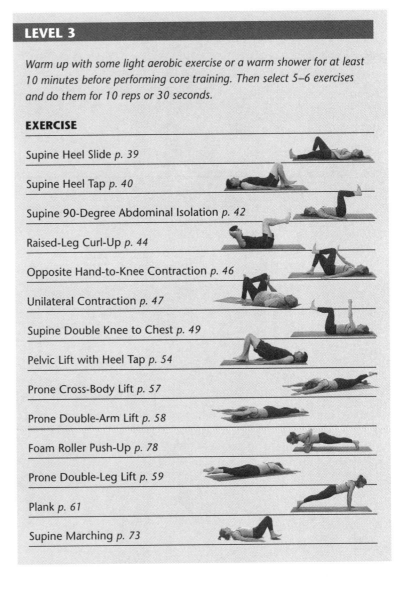

LEVEL 3

Warm up with some light aerobic exercise or a warm shower for at least 10 minutes before performing core training. Then select 5–6 exercises and do them for 10 reps or 30 seconds.

EXERCISE

Supine Heel Slide *p. 39*

Supine Heel Tap *p. 40*

Supine 90-Degree Abdominal Isolation *p. 42*

Raised-Leg Curl-Up *p. 44*

Opposite Hand-to-Knee Contraction *p. 46*

Unilateral Contraction *p. 47*

Supine Double Knee to Chest *p. 49*

Pelvic Lift with Heel Tap *p. 54*

Prone Cross-Body Lift *p. 57*

Prone Double-Arm Lift *p. 58*

Foam Roller Push-Up *p. 78*

Prone Double-Leg Lift *p. 59*

Plank *p. 61*

Supine Marching *p. 73*

level 3 continued

EXERCISE

Ball Sit with Hip Movement *p. 86*

Ball Sit with Foot Lift *p. 87*

Ball Sit with Leg Extension *p. 88*

Ball Sit with Leg Extension & Arm Lift *p. 89*

Supine Base Position on Ball *p. 90*

Prone Arm Raise on Ball *p. 96*

Prone Leg Raise on Ball *p. 97*

Prone Arm & Leg Raise on Ball *p. 98*

Ball Crunch *p. 91*

Twisting Ball Crunch *p. 92*

Reverse Trunk Curl on Ball *p. 93*

Ball Roll-In *p. 94*

Ball Pelvic Lift *p. 95*

Prone Torso Extension on Ball *p. 99*

Ball Wall Slide *p. 102*

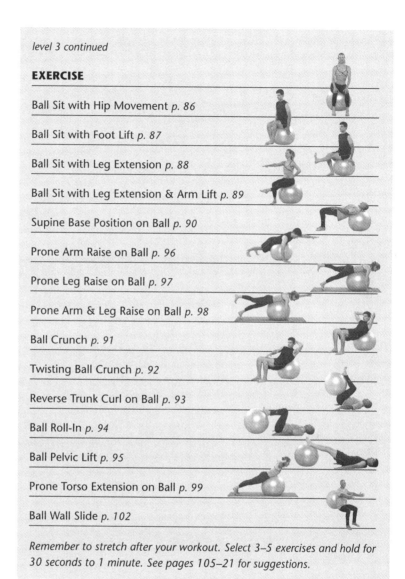

Remember to stretch after your workout. Select 3–5 exercises and hold for 30 seconds to 1 minute. See pages 105–21 for suggestions.

level 4

This super-advanced program is designed for the highly motivated. It's extremely challenging and also includes some fun partner moves.

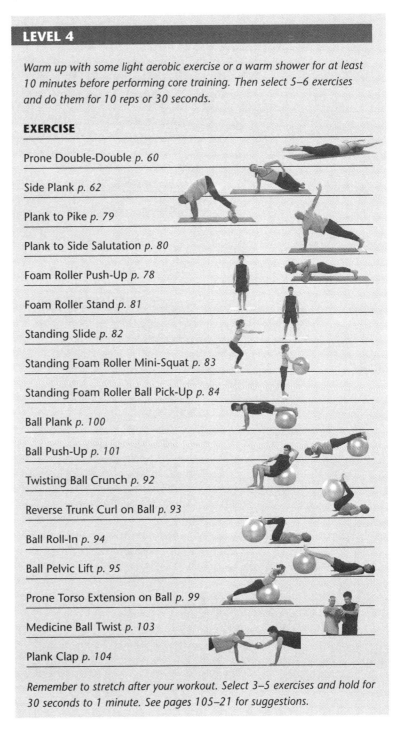

LEVEL 4

Warm up with some light aerobic exercise or a warm shower for at least 10 minutes before performing core training. Then select 5–6 exercises and do them for 10 reps or 30 seconds.

EXERCISE

Prone Double-Double *p. 60*

Side Plank *p. 62*

Plank to Pike *p. 79*

Plank to Side Salutation *p. 80*

Foam Roller Push-Up *p. 78*

Foam Roller Stand *p. 81*

Standing Slide *p. 82*

Standing Foam Roller Mini-Squat *p. 83*

Standing Foam Roller Ball Pick-Up *p. 84*

Ball Plank *p. 100*

Ball Push-Up *p. 101*

Twisting Ball Crunch *p. 92*

Reverse Trunk Curl on Ball *p. 93*

Ball Roll-In *p. 94*

Ball Pelvic Lift *p. 95*

Prone Torso Extension on Ball *p. 99*

Medicine Ball Twist *p. 103*

Plank Clap *p. 104*

Remember to stretch after your workout. Select 3–5 exercises and hold for 30 seconds to 1 minute. See pages 105–21 for suggestions.

part 3

the
exercises

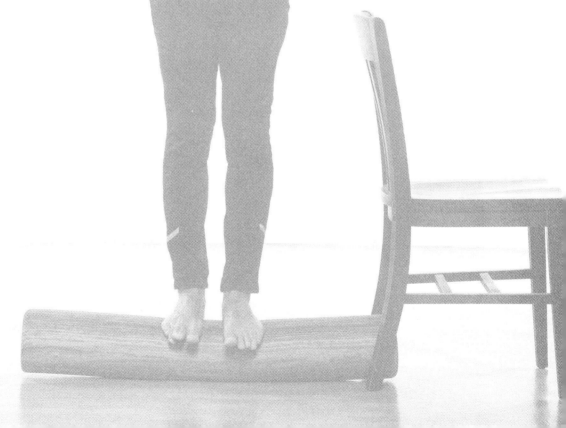

The purpose of this exercise is to gain awareness of core muscles, braced breathing, and proper posture, with the long-term goal of teaching you to be able to locate a neutral spine position with the least amount of effort in any position.

STARTING POSITION: Lie on your back with your knees bent and feet flat on the floor.

START

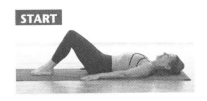

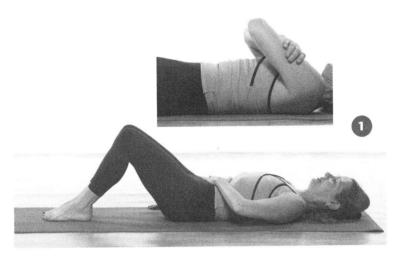

1 Placing one hand on your abs, draw your belly button in as you push the small of your back into the floor. Pretend that you have a sponge in the small of your back and are trying to compress the sponge. Hold for 1–2 seconds.

2 Release and allow the small of your back to return to a comfortable position (arms crossed to show space beneath the low back).

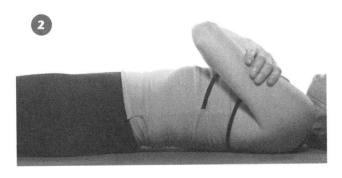

VARIATIONS: You may place your fingers under the small of your back to better feel the move. If it's uncomfortable to place your head on the floor, place a small pillow under your head at first.

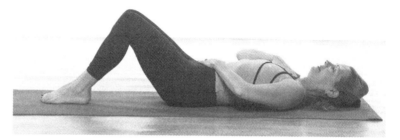

BREATHING OPTION 1 (DIAPHRAGMATIC BREATHING):
Place one hand on your belly and the other hand on your chest. Slowly breathe in through your nose for a count of 1-2-3-4, hold for 4 counts, and then slowly exhale via pursed lips for a count of 4. Repeat several times.

BREATHING OPTION 2 (BRACED BREATHING): Pretend you're about to be punched in the belly and hold that position for 1–5 seconds and perform slow diaphragmatic breathing. This concept is useful to learn for when doing moderately heavy lifts. It will increase intra-abdominal pressure and may provide some level of stabilization.

While this may appear to be a leg exercise, it emphasizes the engagement of the abdominal muscles.

STARTING POSITION: Lie on your back with your knees bent and feet flat on the floor. Find and maintain neutral spine position and place a tennis ball between your knees. Extend your arms along your sides.

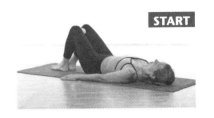

START

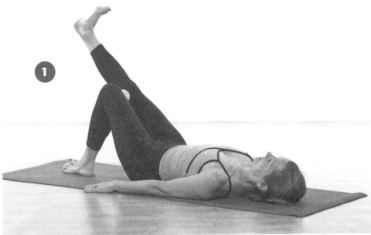

1

1 Keeping the tennis ball in place, slowly and purposefully extend your right leg from the knee joint and flex your foot. Mindfully engage your abs while performing the leg movement. Avoid rapid leg motions and keep the arch in your back to a minimum.

2 Slowly return to the starting position.

Reposition into proper neutral spine position and switch legs.

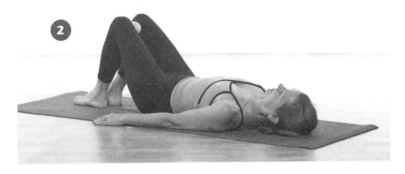

2

This exercise will help you maintain neutral position while moving your extremities.

STARTING POSITION: Lie on your back with your knees bent and feet flat on the floor; find and maintain neutral spine position. Extend both arms directly above your shoulders with your palms facing each other.

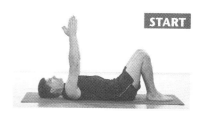

START

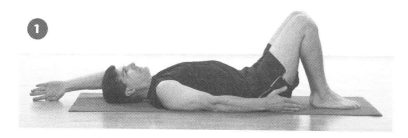

1 Keeping your arms somewhat straight, slowly move one arm forward (lead with the pinky) toward your hip and the other back toward your ear (lead with the thumb).

2 Slowly return to starting position and then move the arms the other direction.

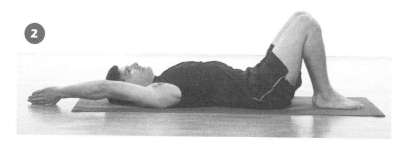

VARIATIONS: Swing both arms back, both arms to the front, and both arms to the sides.

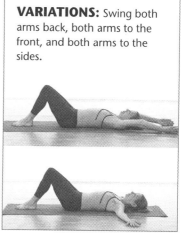

This exercise teaches neutral spine position and conditions the abdominal region. Pelvic control is critical in this exercise. Speed is not important, nor is the number of repetitions. Do not perform this move until you can perform the Supine Leg Extension (page 36) and Supine Arm Swing (page 37) correctly. In addition, if your low back arch increases, you're not ready for this exercise; continue working on the previous exercises.

STARTING POSITION: Lie on your back with your knees bent and feet flat on the floor; find and maintain neutral spine position. Keeping your knees together, extend both arms directly above your shoulders with your palms facing each other.

START

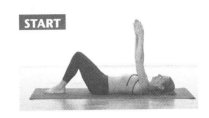

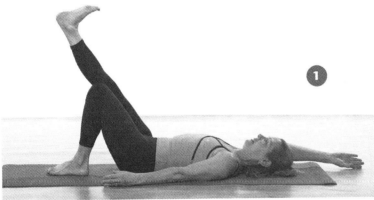

1 Slowly move your right arm back toward your ear and your left arm toward your hip, and simultaneously extend your right leg.

2 Slowly return to starting position and then repeat with the opposite side.

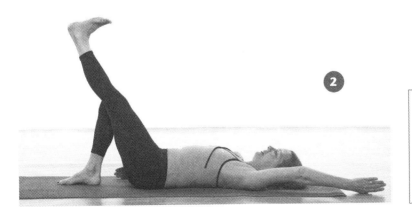

VARIATION: You can also extend the opposite arm and leg (e.g., right leg extends while left arm moves to the ear and right arm moves to the hip).

This exercise teaches core stabilization. Do not allow your low back to arch. It's easier to perform on a smooth floor with stocking feet.

STARTING POSITION: Lie on your back with your knees bent and feet flat on the floor; find and maintain neutral spine position. You may place your hands on your abs to remind yourself to engage them throughout the movement.

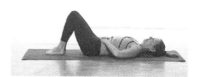

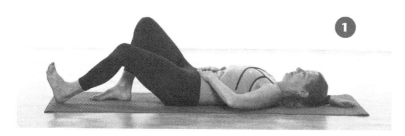

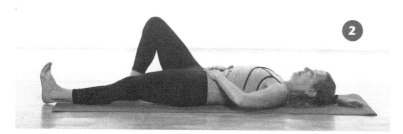

1–2 Keeping your core engaged, slowly and mindfully slide your left heel forward along the floor. Only move your heel out as far as you can while still keeping your low back neutral.

Return to starting position and then slide the right heel out.

This exercise teaches core stabilization and conditions the abdominal region. Do not allow your low back to arch.

STARTING POSITION: Lie on your back with your knees bent and feet flat on the floor; find and maintain neutral spine position. Extend your arms along your sides.

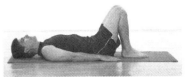

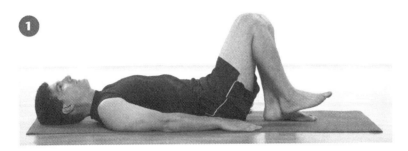

1 Slowly lift your right heel 1–3 inches off the floor. Only lift your heel as high as you can while still keeping neutral spine position. Periodically touch your abdominal muscles to make sure that you're engaging them.

2 Slowly return your heel to the floor, reposition your spine, and repeat with your left heel.

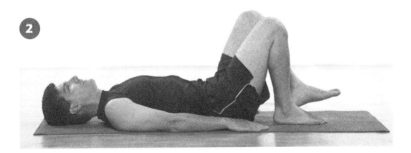

supine foot press

This exercise conditions the abdominal region and teaches core stabilization. Do not allow your low back to arch.

STARTING POSITION: Lie on your back with your knees bent and feet flat on the floor; find and maintain neutral spine position. Raise both legs to a 90-degree angle, as if resting your lower legs on a chair. Extend your arms along your sides. Make sure to maintain proper neutral spine position throughout the exercise.

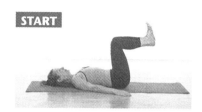
START

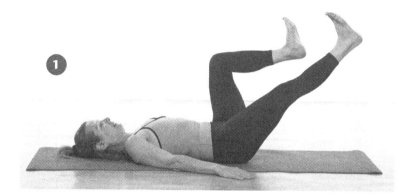

1 Keeping both legs elevated, press your right foot forward and away from you. Only extend your leg as far as you can while still maintaining neutral position.

2 Return to starting position and repeat on the other side.

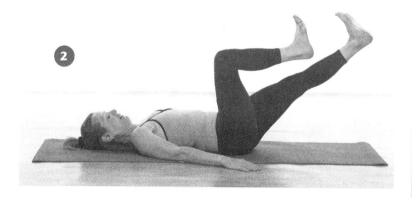

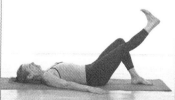
MODIFICATION: You may find it easier to do only one side at a time while keeping the other foot on the floor for better stabilization.

This exercise strengthens and conditions the abdominal muscles while maintaining core stability.

THE POSITION: Lie on your back and lift both legs to 90 degrees. Keep your shoulders on the floor and extend your arms alongside your body. Draw your belly button in and contract your abs hard, as if bearing down. Hold, but don't hold your breath—remember to breathe! Relax and repeat when ready.

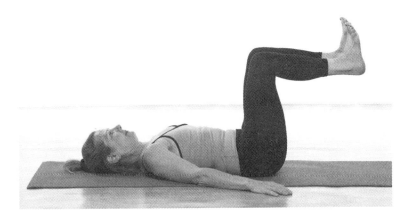

This half sit-up conditions the abdominal region.

STARTING POSITION: Lie on your back with your knees bent and feet flat on the floor; find and maintain neutral spine position. Place your hands behind your head to cradle and support your neck. Tuck your chin to your chest and inhale to begin.

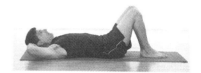

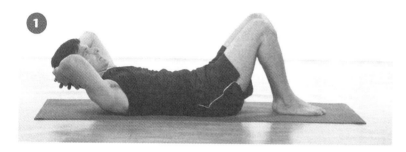

1 While contracting your abdominal muscles, exhale and slowly lift your shoulder blades off the floor. Hold for 1–3 seconds. Don't force yourself to come up higher than is comfortable, and don't use your arms to pull on your neck. Perform this correctly, not quickly.

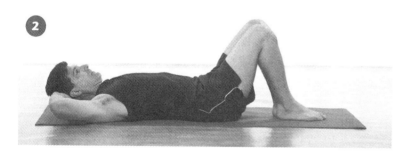

2 Inhale and slowly return to starting position, pressing the small of your back into the floor.

This exercise strengthens and conditions the abdominal region.

STARTING POSITION: Lie on your back, bend your knees 90 degrees, and raise your legs so that your lower legs are parallel to the floor. Find and maintain neutral spine position. Place your hands behind your head to cradle and support your neck. Tuck your chin to your chest and inhale to begin.

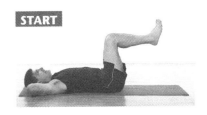
START

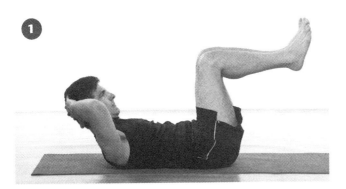
1

1 While contracting your abdominal muscles, exhale and slowly lift your shoulder blades off the floor. Focus on pressing your low back into the floor. Hold for 1–3 seconds. Don't force yourself to come up higher than is comfortable, and don't use your arms to pull on your neck. Perform this correctly, not quickly.

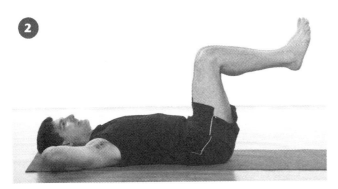
2

2 Inhale and slowly return to starting position, pressing the small of your back into the floor.

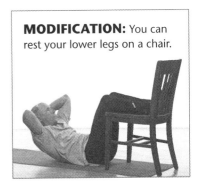
MODIFICATION: You can rest your lower legs on a chair.

This exercise strengthens and conditions the abdominal region.

CAUTION: Do not perform this exercise if rotation aggravates your back.

STARTING POSITION: Lie on your back with your knees bent and feet flat on the floor; find and maintain neutral spine position. Place your hands behind your head to cradle and support your neck. Tuck your chin to your chest and inhale to begin.

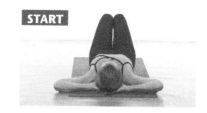

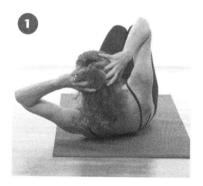

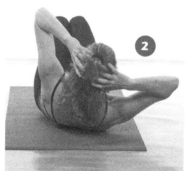

1 While contracting your abdominal muscles, exhale and slowly lift your shoulder blades off the floor, then gently twist your right elbow toward your left knee. Don't force it! Focus on pressing your low back into the floor. Hold for 1–3 seconds.

2 Inhale and slowly return to starting position, then repeat to the opposite side.

VARIATION: For an extra challenge, bend your knees 90 degrees and raise your legs so that your lower legs are parallel to the floor.

This exercise strengthens and conditions the abdominal region.

CAUTION: Avoid this exercise if you have high blood pressure.

STARTING POSITION: Lie on your back with your knees bent and feet flat on the floor; find and maintain neutral spine position.

START

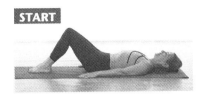

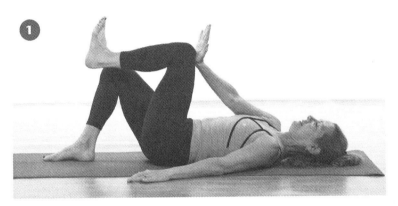

1 Raise your left knee to 90 degrees and place your right hand on your left knee. Keeping your arm straight, press your hand into your knee while simultaneously pressing your knee into your hand. Release after a count of 2. This is an isometric contraction. Feel the abdominal muscles engage. Do not hold your breath. The focus is on pressing your low back into the floor.

Repeat and then switch sides.

This exercise strengthens and conditions the abdominal region.

CAUTION: Avoid this exercise if you have high blood pressure.

STARTING POSITION: Lie on your back with your knees bent and feet flat on the floor; find and maintain neutral spine position.

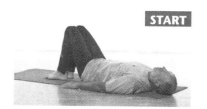

START

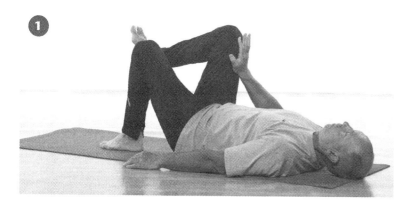

1

1 Raise your right knee to 90 degrees and place your right hand on the knee. Keeping your arm straight, press your right hand into your right knee. Release after a count of 2. This is an isometric contraction. Feel the abdominal muscles engage. Do not hold your breath. The focus is on pressing your low back into the floor.

Repeat and then switch sides.

This exercise strengthens and conditions the abdominal region.

CAUTION: Avoid this exercise if twisting bothers your back.

STARTING POSITION: Lie on your back with your knees bent and feet flat on the floor. Place your hands behind your head. Find and maintain neutral spine position. Inhale and tuck your chin to your chest.

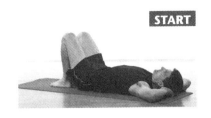
START

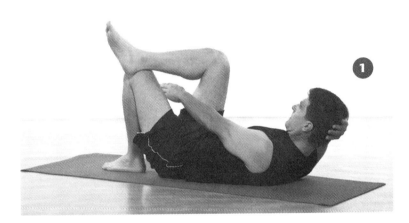
1

1 Place your right ankle on your left knee. Exhale and extend your left hand between the open space of your legs while contracting your abdominal muscles to slowly lift your shoulder blades off the floor while gently twisting your torso to the right. Focus on pressing your low back into the floor. Don't use your arms to pull on your neck. Hold for 1–3 seconds.

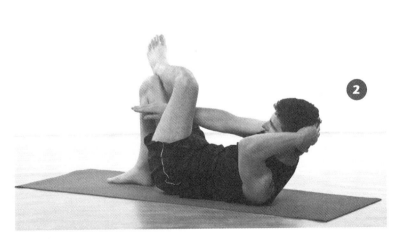
2

2 Slowly return your shoulders to the floor and repeat on the same side before switching sides.

THE POSITION: Lie on your back with your knees bent and feet flat on the floor; find and maintain neutral spine position. Keeping your tailbone down, bring your knees to a 90-degree angle and extend your arms toward the ceiling. Contract the abdominal region to slowly lift your knees 1–3 inches upward. The motion is almost unnoticeable. Do not hold your breath. Relax.

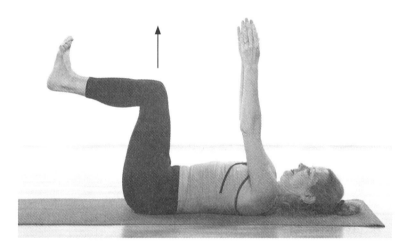

This exercise strengthens the abdominal muscles, buttocks, and low back. Focus on using your gluteals rather than your hamstrings.

CAUTION: Be careful not to perform so many reps that you trigger a hamstring cramp.

STARTING POSITION: Lie on your back with your knees bent and feet flat on the floor; extend your arms alongside your body. Find and maintain neutral spine position.

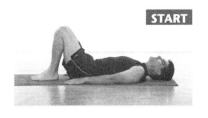
START

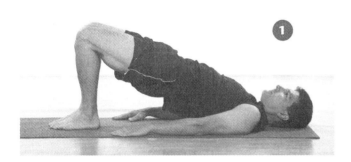
1

1 Pressing both feet equally into the floor, tuck your tailbone between your legs and squeeze your gluteal muscles to lift your butt off the floor. Do not lift your butt so high that it arches your back. Hold for 3–5 seconds.

2 Slowly lower to the floor. Realign your spine after each rep.

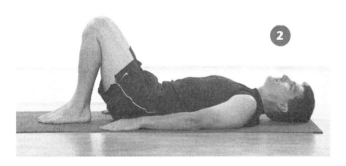
2

This exercise strengthens the abdominal muscles, buttocks, and low back.

CAUTION: Be careful not to perform so many reps that you trigger a hamstring cramp.

STARTING POSITION: Lie on your back with your knees bent and feet flat on the floor. Locate and maintain neutral spine position. Extend your arms along your sides.

START

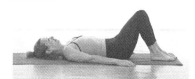

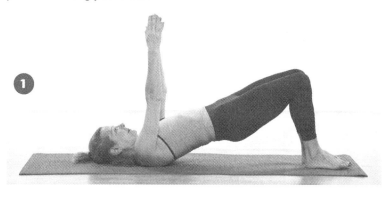

1 Pressing both feet equally into the floor, tuck your tailbone between your legs and squeeze your gluteal muscles to lift your butt off the floor. Do not lift your butt so high that it arches your back. Once you're in a comfortable position, raise your arms straight up toward the ceiling with your palms facing each other.

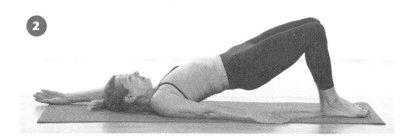

2 Keeping your core engaged and both arms straight, slowly move one arm forward toward the hip and the other hand back toward the ear.

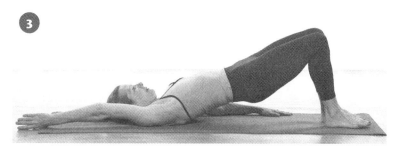

3 Continue alternating arms, making sure to realign your spine after each rep.

Once you've completed the desired number of reps, slowly lower your rear end to the floor.

While this exercise may appear to be a leg exercise, it emphasizes low back muscle engagement and strengthens the abdominal muscles, buttocks, and low back.

STARTING POSITION: Lie on your back with your knees bent and feet flat on the floor. Find and maintain neutral spine position, then place a tennis ball between your knees. Extend your arms alongside your body. Pressing both feet equally into the floor, tuck your tailbone between your legs and squeeze your gluteal muscles to lift your butt off the floor.

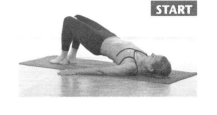

START

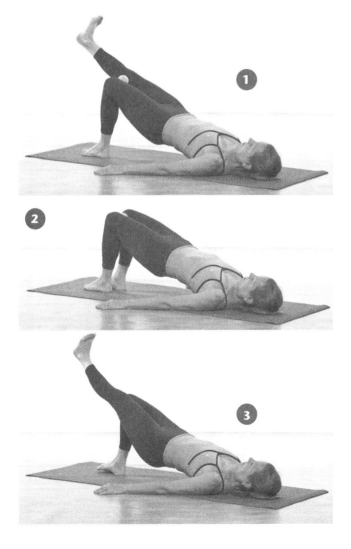

1 Keeping the tennis ball in place, slowly and purposefully extend your right leg from the knee joint. Mindfully engage your abdomen and gluteal muscles. Avoid rapid leg motions.

2 Slowly return to starting position and reposition into proper neutral spine position if necessary.

3 Perform with the left leg.

This exercise strengthens the abdominal muscles, buttocks, and low back. Make sure you can perform Pelvic Lift with Arm Lift (page 51) and Pelvic Lift with Leg Extension (page 52) correctly before trying this combination exercise.

STARTING POSITION: Lie on your back with your knees bent and feet flat on the floor. Find and maintain neutral spine position, then place a tennis ball between your knees. Extend both arms straight up to the ceiling, with your palms facing each other. Pressing both feet equally into the floor, tuck your tailbone between your legs and squeeze your gluteal muscles to lift your butt off the floor.

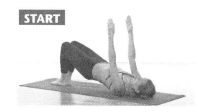

START

1 Keeping the tennis ball in place, slowly extend your left leg from the knee joint while your left arm moves toward your hip and your right arm moves back toward your ear. Mindfully engage the butt muscles while performing the leg movement.

2 Slowly return to starting position.

3 Reposition into proper neutral spine position and then perform on the other side.

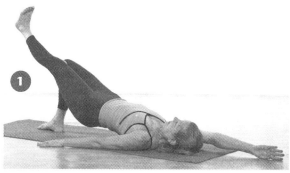

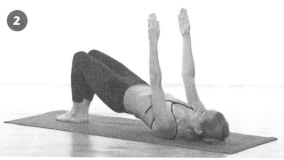

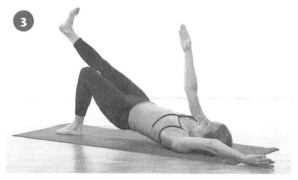

This exercise strengthens the abdominal muscles, buttocks, and low back. Periodically touch your butt muscles to make sure that you're engaging them.

STARTING POSITION: Lie on your back with your knees bent and feet flat on the floor. Find and maintain neutral spine position, then extend your arms alongside your body. Pressing both feet equally into the floor, tuck your tailbone under and squeeze your gluteal muscles to lift your butt off the floor. Hold for 3–5 seconds.

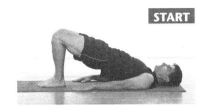
START

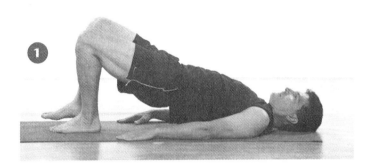

1 Slowly lift your right heel 1–3 inches off the floor.

2 Slowly return your heel to the floor and reposition your spine.

3 Perform with your left heel.

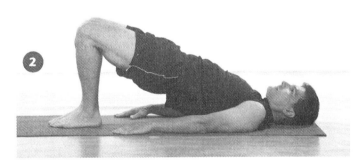

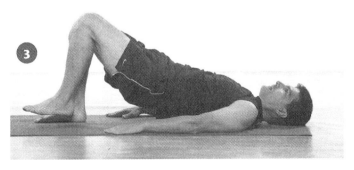

This exercise strengthens your lower spine muscles as well as your gluteals. Some people find it more comfortable to place a rolled-up towel or pillow under the hipbones when doing this. Your body will tell you if you need a pillow under your hips.

CAUTION: Do not perform this exercise if you find arching your back uncomfortable.

STARTING POSITION: Lie face-down with your arms outstretched so that your biceps are next to your ears and your palms are down.

START

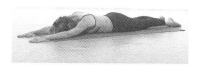

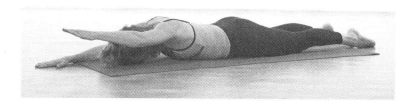

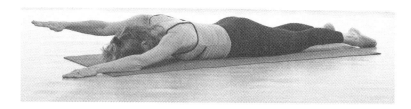

1 Concentrating on maintaining correct alignment (this means no excessive arching of your back), slowly raise one arm to a comfortable height and hold. Do not raise the arm so high that you cause your back to arch! Keep the motion smooth and avoid twisting your body.

2 Lower the arm and raise the other arm and hold.

MODIFICATION: If your shoulders are inflexible, place your arms alongside your body or turn your thumb up while raising the arm.

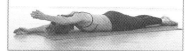

This exercise strengthens your lower spine muscles as well as your gluteals. Some people find it more comfortable to place a rolled-up towel or pillow under the hipbones when doing this. Your body will tell you if you need a pillow under your hips.

CAUTION: If you feel an uncomfortable sensation in your low back, stop!

STARTING POSITION: Lie face-down with your arms outstretched so that your biceps are next to your ears and your palms are down.

START

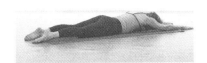

1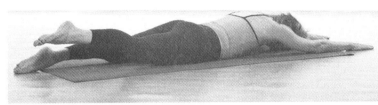

1 Concentrating on maintaining correct alignment (this means no excessive arching of your back), slowly raise one leg a comfortable height and hold for 1–3 seconds. Keep the motion smooth and avoid twisting your body.

2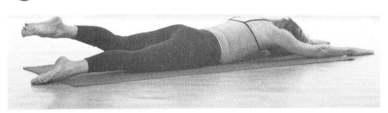

2 Lower the leg and raise the other leg and hold.

MODIFICATION: If your shoulders are inflexible, place your arms alongside your body or turn your thumbs up.

This exercise strengthens your lower spine muscles as well as your gluteals. Some people find it more comfortable to place a rolled-up towel or pillow under the hipbones when doing this. Your body will tell you if you need a pillow under your hips.

CAUTION: If you feel an uncomfortable sensation in your low back, stop!

STARTING POSITION: Lie face-down with your arms outstretched so that your biceps are next to your ears and your palms are down.

START

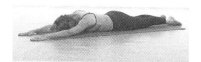

1

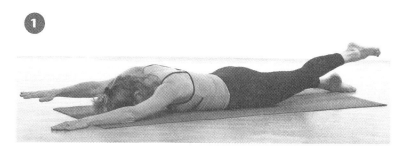

2

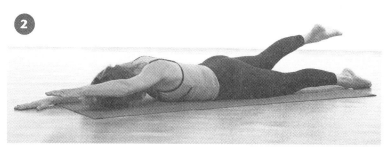

1 Concentrating on maintaining correct alignment (this means no excessive arching of your back), slowly raise your right arm and your left leg a comfortable height and hold for 1–3 seconds. Your foot shouldn't raise up much higher than your rear end. Keep the motion smooth and avoid twisting your body.

2 Lower your arm and leg, and then raise the opposite arm and leg. Hold.

MODIFICATION: If your shoulders are inflexible, turn your thumb up while raising your arm.

This advanced exercise strengthens your lower spine muscles as well as your gluteals. Some people find it more comfortable to place a rolled-up towel or pillow under the hipbones when doing this. Your body will tell you if you need a pillow under your hips.

CAUTION: If you feel an uncomfortable sensation in your low back, stop!

STARTING POSITION: Lie face-down with your arms outstretched so that your biceps are next to your ears and your palms are down.

START

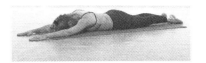

1

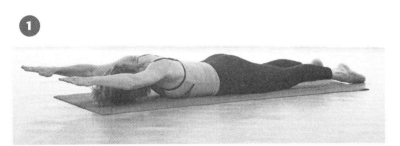

1 Concentrating on maintaining correct alignment (this means no excessive arching of your back), slowly raise both arms and hold for 1–3 seconds. Keep the motion smooth and avoid twisting your body.

2

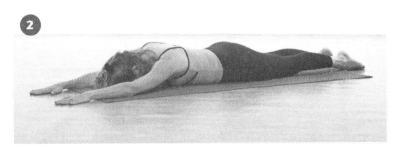

2 Lower your arms and relax.

MODIFICATION: If your shoulders are inflexible, turn your thumbs up while raising your arms.

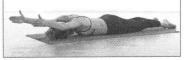

This exercise strengthens your lower spine muscles as well as your gluteals. Some people find it more comfortable to place a rolled-up towel or pillow under the hipbones when doing this. Your body will tell you if you need a pillow under your hips.

CAUTION: If you feel an uncomfortable sensation in your low back, stop!

STARTING POSITION: Lie face-down with your arms outstretched so that your biceps are next to your ears and your palms are down.

START

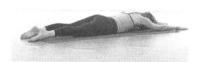

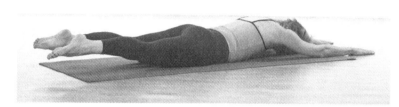

1 Concentrating on maintaining correct alignment (this means no excessive arching of your back), slowly raise both legs and hold for 1–3 seconds. Keep the motion smooth and avoid twisting your body.

2 Lower your legs and relax.

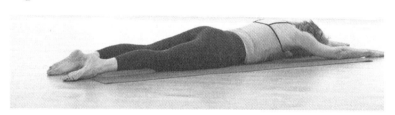

MODIFICATION: If your shoulders are inflexible, place your arms alongside your body or turn your thumbs up.

prone floor series
prone double-double

This exercise strengthens your lower spine muscles as well as your gluteals. Some people find it more comfortable to place a rolled-up towel or pillow under the hipbones when doing this. Your body will tell you if you need a pillow under your hips.

CAUTION: If you feel an uncomfortable sensation in your low back, stop!

STARTING POSITION: Lie face-down with your arms outstretched so that your biceps are next to your ears and your palms are down.

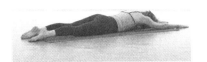

START

1 Concentrating on maintaining correct alignment (this means no excessive arching of your back), slowly raise both arms and legs and hold for 1–3 seconds. Keep the motion smooth and avoid twisting your body.

1

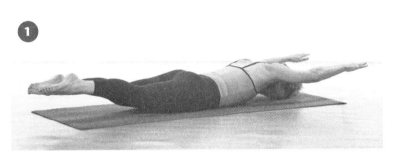

2

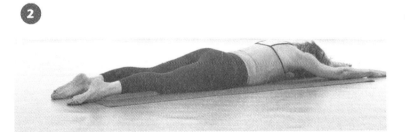

2 Lower your arms and legs and relax.

MODIFICATION: If your shoulders are inflexible, turn your thumbs up while raising the arms.

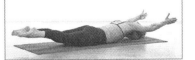

plank

This exercise tones and conditions the entire core. Additionally, it serves as a foundational exercise and screening tool to let you know if you're ready for the foam roller series that starts on page 68. You need to be able to perform the next two exercises perfectly before moving to the foam roller series.

CAUTION: Do not perform this exercise if you have high blood pressure or shoulder joint issues.

THE POSITION: Assume a traditional push-up position, with your hands under your shoulders, arms extended, and your feet extended behind you. Brace your abs so that your back forms a nice line from head to heels—no "sagging" in the middle or piking your butt to the ceiling. Hold for 3 seconds, working toward the goal of 1 minute. Breathe normally.

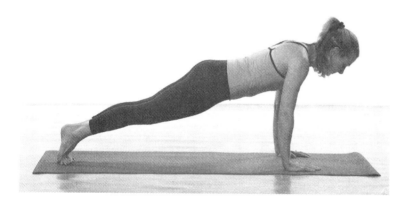

This exercise works the lateral muscles (the quadratus lumborum) of the torso.

CAUTION: Do not perform this exercise if you have high blood pressure or shoulder joint issues.

STARTING POSITION: Lie on your right side with your knees bent, stacking your shoulders, ankles, knees, and hips atop each other.

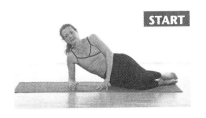
START

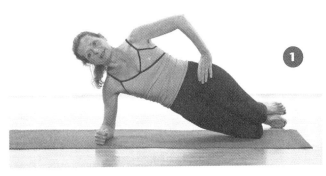
1

1 Balancing on your forearm and lower knee, lift your hips off the floor and straighten yourself up by engaging your entire core. Align your chin, sternum, and mid-pelvic area. Hold. Breathe normally.

2 Lower to starting position.

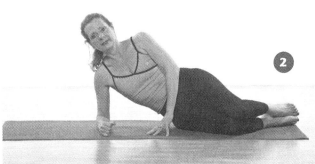
2

VARIATION: If you're very fit, try balancing yourself on your forearm and lower foot or, if super fit, your hand and lower foot.

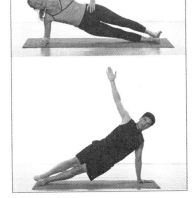

This exercise strengthens your gluteal muscles.

STARTING POSITION: Lie on your left side and pull both knees halfway to your chest, stacking your ankles, knees, and hips atop each other.

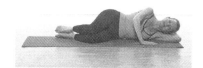

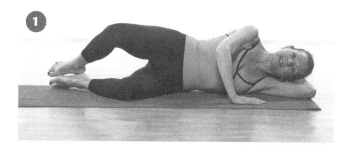

1 Slowly lift your right knee 2–5 inches above the other knee.

2 Lower and repeat.

Once you've finished your prescribed number of reps, roll over and repeat on the other side.

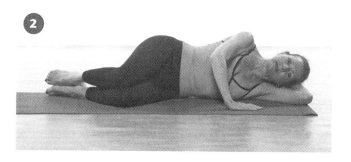

This exercise strengthens the low back muscles and teaches body awareness.

STARTING POSITION: Assume proper tabletop position and find neutral spine. Stabilize your low back by engaging/bracing your abdominal muscles.

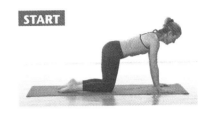

START

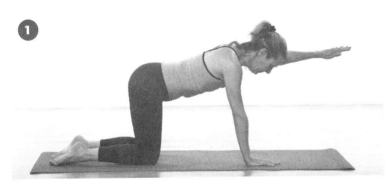

1

1 Keeping your torso steady and the base of your skull in alignment with your spine, raise your left arm to shoulder height or as high as is comfortable. Hold for 1–5 seconds.

2 Lower to starting position and perform with the other arm.

Continue alternating.

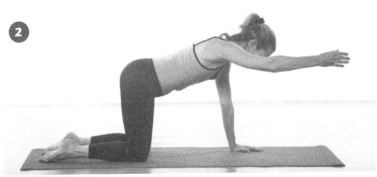

2

This exercise strengthens the low back and gluteal muscles and also teaches body awareness.

STARTING POSITION: Assume proper tabletop position and find neutral spine. Stabilize your low back by engaging/bracing your abdominal muscles.

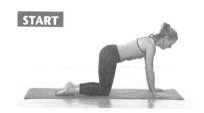

START

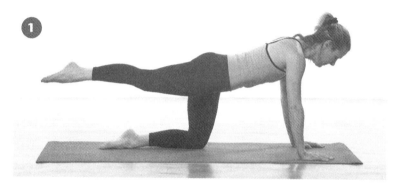

1 Keeping your torso steady and the base of your skull in alignment with your spine, raise your right leg. Hold for 1–5 seconds.

2 Lower to starting position and perform with the other leg.

Continue alternating.

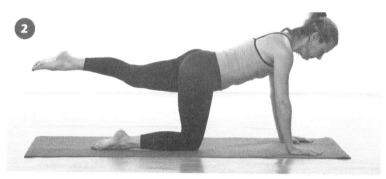

This exercise strengthens the low back and gluteal muscles and also teaches body awareness.

STARTING POSITION: Assume proper tabletop position and find neutral spine. Stabilize your low back by engaging/bracing your abdominal muscles.

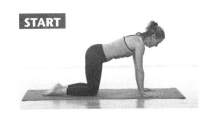

START

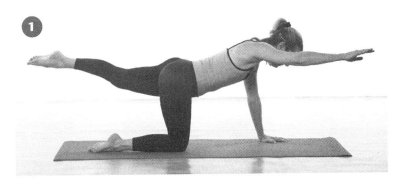

1

1 Keeping your torso steady and the base of your skull in alignment with your spine, raise your right arm and left leg to a comfortable height. Hold for 1–5 seconds.

2 Lower to starting position and perform with your right leg and left arm.

Continue alternating.

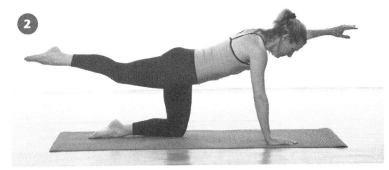

2

This exercise challenges the muscles that maintain core/spinal stabilization. Form and control is critical!

STARTING POSITION: Assume proper tabletop position and find neutral spine. Stabilize your low back by engaging/bracing your abdominal muscles.

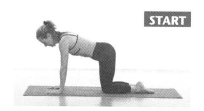

START

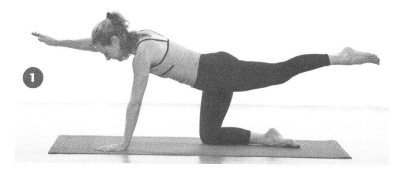

1 Raise your right arm forward and extend your left leg straight behind you and hold for 1–3 seconds.

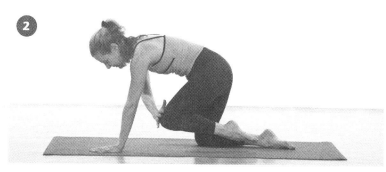

2 Keeping your torso steady and maintaining proper alignment from the base of your skull to your tailbone, bring your right hand toward your left knee and your left knee toward your right hand as they meet under your abdominal region. Hold steady for 1–2 seconds—don't rock!

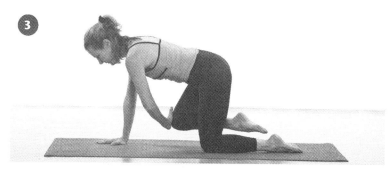

3 Return to starting position, readjust posture, and repeat on the opposite side.

VARIATION: You can also bring your right elbow to your right knee, and then your left elbow to your left knee.

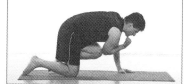

This exercise improves low back range of motion and neutral-spine awareness.

STARTING POSITION: Place a full-length half roller flat-side up across a chair. Sit upright on the roller, with your tailbone off the roller. Let your feet rest on the floor.

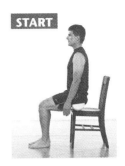

START

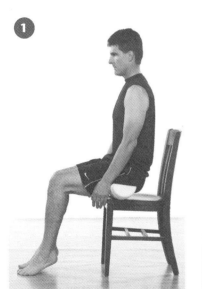

1

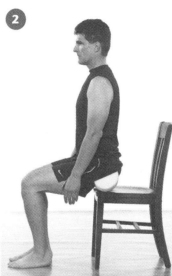

2

1 Slowly roll your tailbone under you.

2 Slowly roll your tailbone backward, allowing your back to arch comfortably.

Continue rolling forward and back mindfully, paying attention to the pelvic position that feels best for you.

This exercise acquaints you with the roller. This is the starting platform for all foam roller exercises. Once you feel safe and comfortable with this exercise, you're ready for the rest of the foam roller series.

STARTING POSITION: Place a full-length roller on the floor and lie on it from head to tailbone. Bend your knees and place your feet on the floor. You may have your arms on the floor to the side for additional stability.

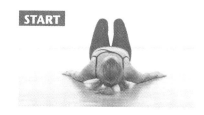

START

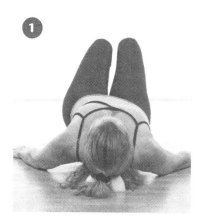

❶

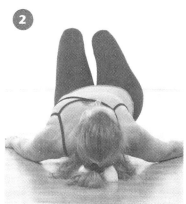

❷

1–2 Once you feel stable, gently rock left and right and recover your balance.

This exercise helps you improve trunk support.

STARTING POSITION: Place a full-length roller on the floor and lie on it from head to tailbone. Bend your knees and place your feet on the floor. Position your arms however you need to for support and balance.

START

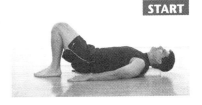

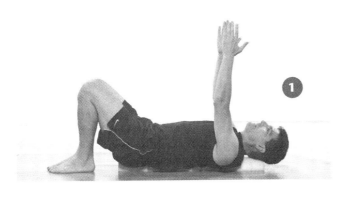

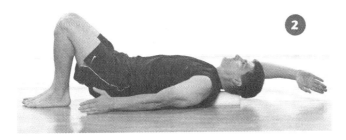

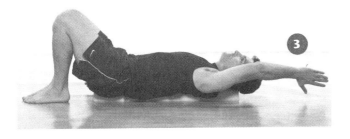

1 Once stable, raise your arms directly above your chest.

2 Now slowly move one arm forward and the other arm back. Try not to fall off the roller.

3 Slowly move the arms in the other direction.

Continue alternating arms.

This exercise helps you gain greater control of your core.

STARTING POSITION: Place a full-length roller on the floor and lie on it from head to tailbone. Bend your knees and place your feet on the floor; place a tennis ball between your knees. Position your arms however you need to for support and balance.

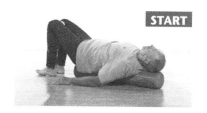

START

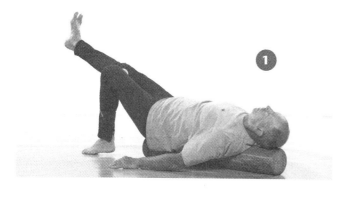

1

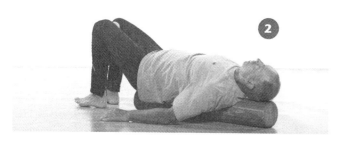

2

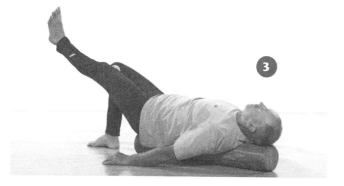

3

1 Once stable, extend your right leg, keeping the ball in place.

2 Lower your leg, making sure to not let the tennis ball drop.

3 Reposition your body and perform the same movement with the other leg.

Continue alternating.

VARIATION: You can also perform the sequence with your arms lifted off the ground or resting across your chest.

This extremely challenging exercise fosters core stabilization.

STARTING POSITION: Place a full-length roller on the floor and lie on it from head to tailbone. Bend your knees and place your feet on the floor; place a tennis ball between your knees. Once stable, raise your arms above your chest.

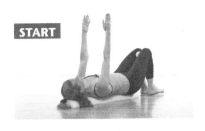

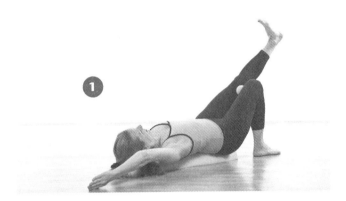

1 Keeping the ball in place, lower your left arm toward your left hip and your right arm back toward your ear as you extend your left leg.

2 Continue alternating.

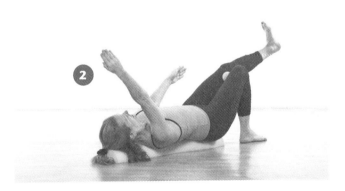

This exercise improves trunk stabilization and abdominal strength.

STARTING POSITION: Place a full-length roller on the floor and lie on it from head to tailbone. Bend your knees and place your feet on the floor. Extend your arms alongside your body for extra support.

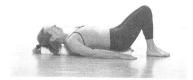

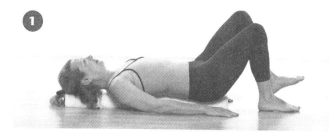

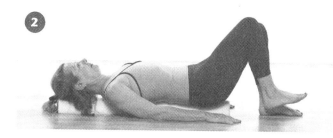

1 Once stable, slowly lift your left foot 1–2 inches off the floor (the less you lift your foot off the floor, the more challenging this exercise is). Hold for 15 seconds. Do not allow your torso or hips to rock.

2 Return to starting position and switch legs.

Continue alternating.

This exercise strengthens the gluteal region and the extensor muscles of the back.

CAUTION: Be careful to avoid hamstring cramps.

STARTING POSITION: Place a full-length roller on the floor and lie on it from head to tailbone. Bend your knees and place your feet on the floor. Extend your arms alongside your body for extra support.

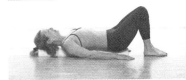

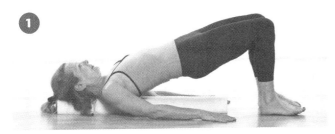

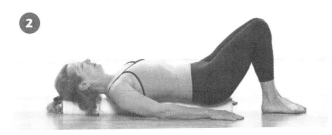

1 Slowly raise your rear end off the roller and hold for 10 seconds. Avoid going too high and arching your back as this can cause cramping of the hamstring muscles.

2 Slowly lower yourself to the roller, realign your spine and repeat.

VARIATION: You can also lie on the floor but place the roller or some other unstable object under your feet to perform the movement. You can also cross your arms across your chest.

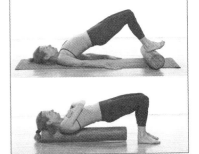

This exercise improves abdominal strength and fosters core stability.

STARTING POSITION: Place a full-length roller on the floor and lie on it from head to tailbone. Bend your knees and place your feet on the floor. Extend your arms alongside your body for extra support.

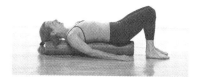

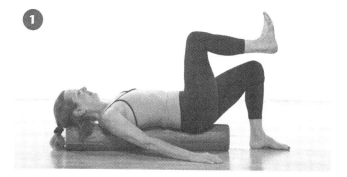

1 Once stable, lift your right leg so that your thigh makes a 90-degree angle with your chest. Hold.

2 Slowly press the leg forward while maintaining proper core stability.

Return to starting position and repeat with the other leg.

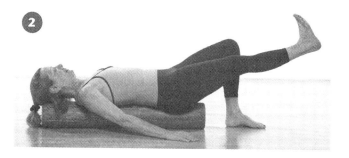

STARTING POSITION: Place a full-length roller under your knees and a second one under your hands.

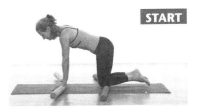

START

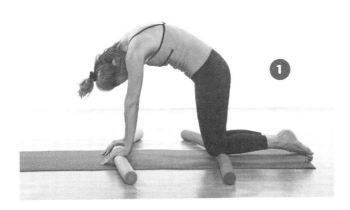

1

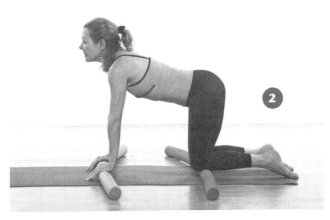

2

1 Inhale and draw your belly in as you round your back.

2 Exhale and arch your back slightly if possible.

This exercise improves core stability and spinal alignment.

CAUTION: Do not progress to this exercise until you can maintain core stabilization in the Mad Cat (page 76).

STARTING POSITION: Place a full-length roller under your knees and a second one under your hands.

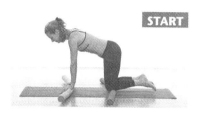

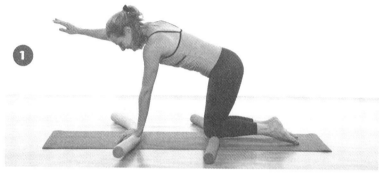

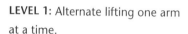

LEVEL 1: Alternate lifting one arm at a time.

LEVEL 2: Alternate lifting one leg at a time.

LEVEL 3: Alternate lifting the opposite arm and leg.

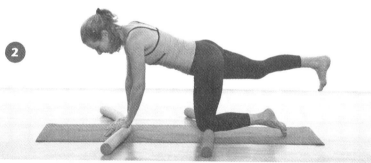

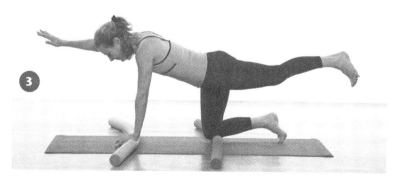

VARIATION: You can also try this with your right hand and knee on one roller, and your left hand and knee on another.

This exercise engages the complete kinetic chain. It's about alignment, not how many push-ups you can do.

STARTING POSITION: Place a full-length roller under your chest and then place your hands shoulder-width apart on top of the roller. Slide your feet back behind you until you're in a high push-up position, with your back forming a straight line from head to heels. Engage your gluteal and abdominal muscles so that you don't sag in the middle.

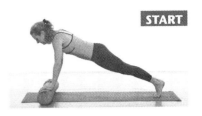

START

1 Keeping your back straight, lower your chest to the roller (or as low as you can) with control.

2 Press back up.

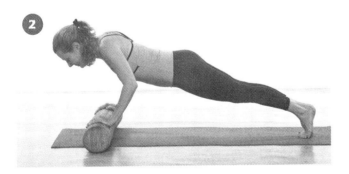

1

2

MODIFICATION: If stability or strength is an issue, you can perform this with your knees on the floor.

VARIATION: Try this with the roller under your feet.

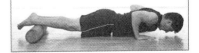

This advanced exercise fosters upper body muscle tone and core stability. Make sure to execute it with proper alignment.

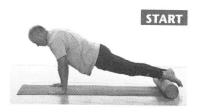

STARTING POSITION: Place a full-length roller under your feet and then place your hands shoulder-width apart on the floor. Slide your feet back behind you until you're in a high push-up position, with your back forming a straight line from head to heels. Maintain this position for 15 seconds.

1

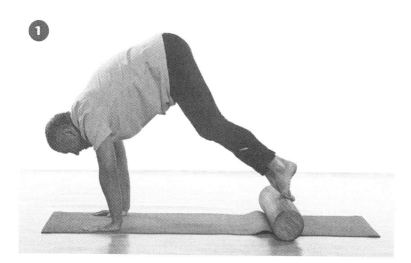

1 Keeping your feet on the roller, roll your feet in toward your hands to lift your rear end up to the ceiling (pike position). Hold.

This extremely advanced exercise fosters upper body muscle tone and core stability.

CAUTION: Avoid this exercise if you have weak shoulders.

STARTING POSITION: Place your toes on a full-length roller and your hands on the floor in a push-up position. Make sure your back forms a straight line from head to heels. Maintain this position for 15 seconds.

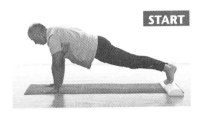
START

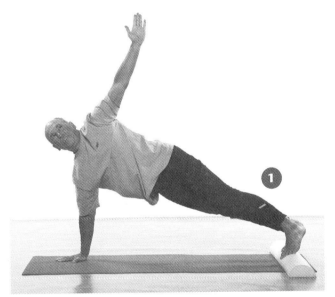

1 Keeping your toes on the roller, slowly rotate your body to the left, relying on your right arm to support you. Extend your left arm to the ceiling so that you're in a side plank.

2 Return to starting position.

Perform on the other side.

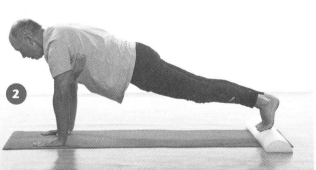

This exercise fosters core stability and balance. If you can't stand on the roller, it's suggested that you return to the seated ball exercises (starting on page 85).

STARTING POSITION: Place a full-length half roller horizontally on the floor in front of you with the flat side down.

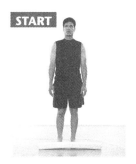

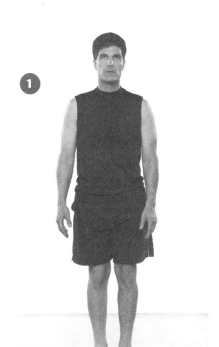

1 Step onto the roller with your left foot and then your right foot, with your feet comfortably apart. Maintain proper posture and hold.

VARIATION: Flip the roller over and perform the exercise with the flat side up, or stand on a circular roller with a chair or wall nearby for support.

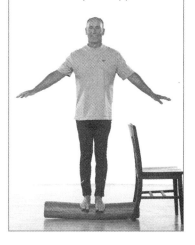

This exercise improves balance and dynamic core stability.

CAUTION: If you can't do the Foam Roller Stand (page 81) with proper posture, do not attempt this exercise.

STARTING POSITION: Place a full-length half roller horizontally on the floor in front of you with the flat side down. Step onto the roller.

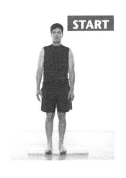

START

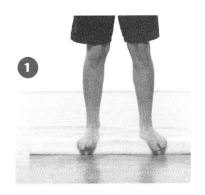

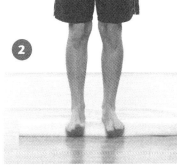

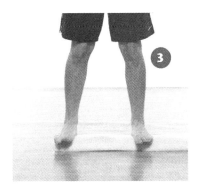

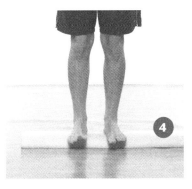

1 Slowly slide your left foot farther to the left and hold.

2 Slowly return your left foot to starting position and hold.

3 Slowly slide your right foot farther to the right and hold.

4 Slowly return your right foot to starting position and hold.

As you advance, move the foot farther toward the end of the roller.

VARIATION: For an extra challenge, try this move with the flat side up.

This exercise improves balance and dynamic core stability and stamina.

CAUTION: If you can't do the Foam Roller Stand (page 81) with proper posture, do not attempt this exercise.

STARTING POSITION: Place a full-length half roller horizontally on the floor in front of you with the flat side down. You may position yourself close to a wall for support. Step onto the roller.

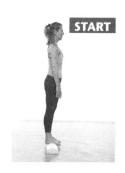

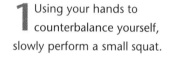

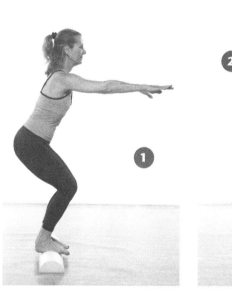

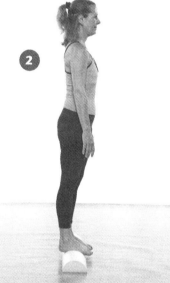

1 Using your hands to counterbalance yourself, slowly perform a small squat.

2 Return to starting position.

VARIATION: As you improve, try crossing your arms or performing the move with the rounded side down.

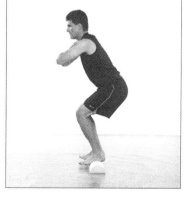

This exercise fosters better balance and core stability.

CAUTION: If you can't do the Foam Roller Stand (page 81) with proper posture, do not attempt this exercise.

STARTING POSITION: Place a full-length half roller horizontally on the floor in front of you with the flat side down. Place a large object such as a big stability ball in front of you. Step onto the roller.

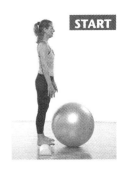
START

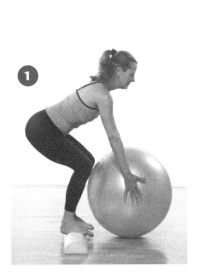

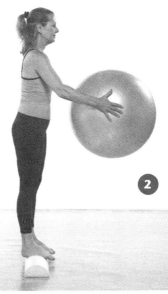

1 Standing in your most stable position, slowly bend down to pick up the object.

2 Return to standing.

This exercise teaches you how to contract your abdominal wall and maintain neutral spine on an unstable surface. This exercise should become so natural that you perform it anytime when sitting in a chair.

THE POSITION: Sit on the ball and find neutral lumbar spine position. Gently engage your abdominal wall muscles. Focus on proper sitting alignment—imagine your head is being lifted up by a string; keep your chest up and out and your shoulder blades together. Hold, then relax.

Continue performing this, each time trying to increase the duration of the hold up to 1 minute.

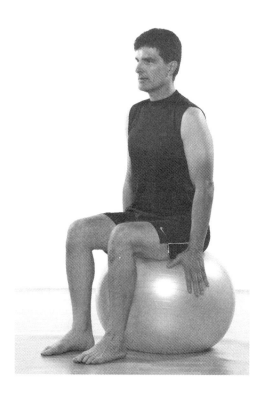

ball sit with hip movement

Do not do the other exercises in this series until you can perform this correctly.

STARTING POSITION: Sit on the ball and find neutral lumbar spine position.

START

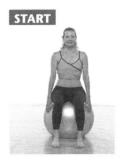

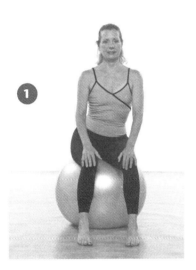

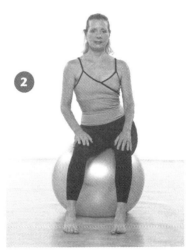

1–2 Using your hips, gently roll the ball from side to side.

3 Roll your tailbone under you to round your low back.

4 Roll your tailbone backward and allow your low back to curve/arch.

Finally, circle your weight in a clockwise direction, then switch directions.

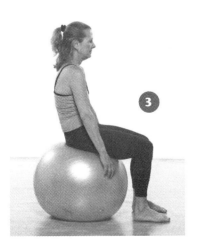

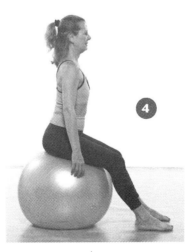

This exercise teaches you how to contract the abdominal wall and maintain neutral spine on an unstable surface. It'll also progressively challenge your system.

STARTING POSITION: Sit on the ball and locate neutral spine position. Gently engage your abdominal wall muscles. Focus on proper sitting alignment—imagine your head is being lifted up by a string; keep your chest up and out and your shoulder blades together.

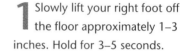

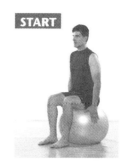

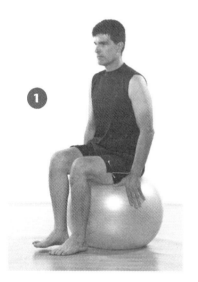

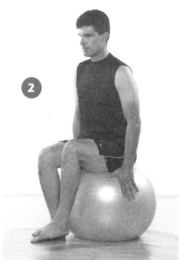

1 Slowly lift your right foot off the floor approximately 1–3 inches. Hold for 3–5 seconds.

2 Slowly lower your foot to the floor and then alternate foot lifts.

MODIFICATION: You can try this while sitting in a chair before progressing to an exercise ball.

This exercise teaches you how to contract the abdominal wall while maintaining neutral spine on an unstable surface. It'll also progressively challenge your system.

STARTING POSITION: Sit on the ball and locate neutral spine position. Gently engage your abdominal wall muscles. Focus on proper sitting alignment—imagine your head is being lifted up by a string; keep your chest up and out and your shoulder blades together.

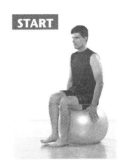

START

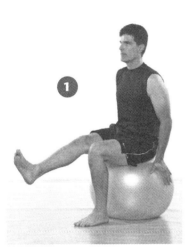

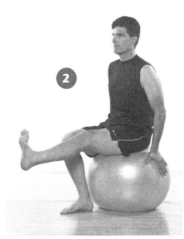

1 Slowly lift your right foot off the floor and extend your leg from the knee joint. Avoid rolling or rocking your pelvic joint. Hold for 3–5 seconds.

2 Slowly lower your foot to the floor and repeat with your other leg.

Continue alternating.

MODIFICATION: You can try this while sitting in a chair before progressing to an exercise ball.

This exercise teaches you how to contract the abdominal wall while maintaining neutral spine on an unstable surface. It'll also progressively challenge your system.

STARTING POSITION: Sit on the ball and locate neutral spine position. Gently engage your abdominal wall muscles. Focus on proper sitting alignment—imagine your head is being lifted up by a string; keep your chest up and out and your shoulder blades together.

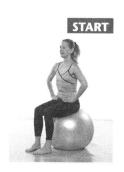
START

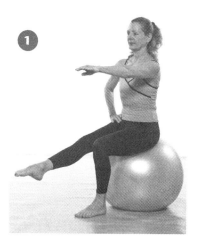

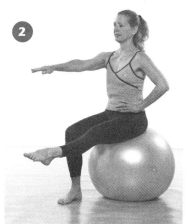

1 Slowly lift your right foot off the floor, extend your leg from the knee joint, and raise your left arm forward. Avoid rolling or rocking your pelvic joint. Hold for 3–5 seconds.

2 Slowly lower your foot to the floor and repeat with your other leg and arm.

Continue alternating.

MODIFICATION: You can try this while sitting in a chair before progressing to an exercise ball.

ball series
supine base position on ball

This exercise teaches you how to contract the abdominal wall and low back muscles and maintain neutral spine on an unstable surface in a supine position. It'll also progressively challenge your system.

STARTING POSITION: Sit on the ball and locate neutral spine position. Gently engage your abdominal wall muscles. Focus on proper sitting alignment—imagine your head is being lifted up by a string; keep your chest up and out and your shoulder blades together.

START

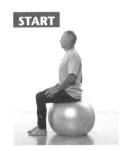

1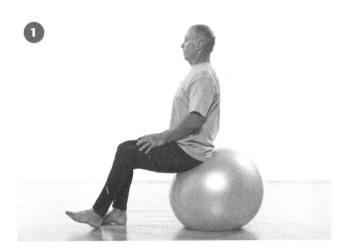

2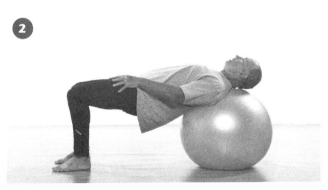

1–2 Slowly walk your feet forward as far as possible, allowing the ball to roll into your mid-back and then the neck region, to form a tabletop position. Hold.

Return to starting position and relax.

MODIFICATION: If you don't have enough core control to move back up the ball, just drop your butt to the floor between each repetition.

This exercise engages the abdominal muscles as well as the internal and external obliques.

STARTING POSITION: Sit on the ball and then slowly walk your feet forward, letting the ball roll beneath you, until you're reclining on the ball with the ball pressed comfortably into your low back. Locate and maintain neutral spine position and then place your hands behind your head. Your knees should be bent 90 degrees and your feet should be on the floor shoulder-width apart.

START

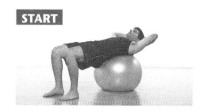

1 Slowly perform a half sit-up by bending at your waist to bring your chest toward your knees.

2 Slowly lower to starting position.

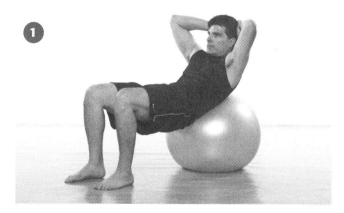

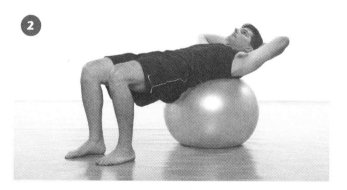

MODIFICATION: For additional stability, move your feet farther away from the ball and spread your feet farther apart.

VARIATION: For an extra balance challenge, place your feet closer together as well as closer to the ball.

ONE-LEG VARIATION: Try performing the crunch while lifting one leg and extending it.

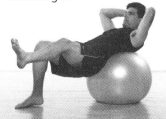

twisting ball crunch

This exercise engages the internal and external obliques.

CAUTION: Do not perform this exercise if rotation bothers your back.

STARTING POSITION: Sit on the ball and then slowly walk your feet forward, letting the ball roll beneath your low back until you're reclining on the ball with the ball pressed comfortably into your low back. Locate and maintain neutral spine position and then place both hands behind your head. Your knees should be bent approximately 90 degrees and your feet should be on the floor shoulder-width apart. Always keep your knees aligned over your ankles.

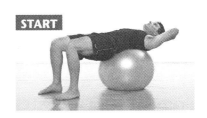

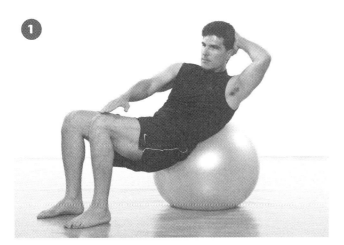

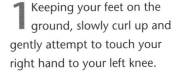 Keeping your feet on the ground, slowly curl up and gently attempt to touch your right hand to your left knee.

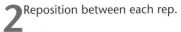 Reposition between each rep.

After you've completed your reps on one side, return to starting position, locate neutral spine position, and perform on the opposite side.

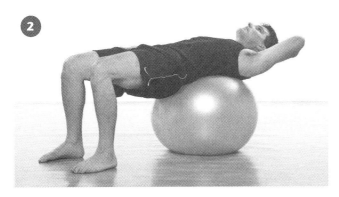

This exercise conditions the abdominal muscles. It's a very advanced exercise—proceed with caution.

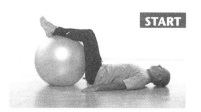

STARTING POSITION: Lie on the floor on your back with your lower legs resting on the exercise ball and knees bent 90 degrees. Extend your arms alongside your body.

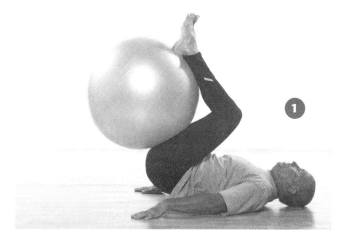

1 Digging your heels into the ball and gripping the ball between your heels and the backs of your thighs, slowly rock/tilt/lift your tailbone off the floor 1–2 inches if possible.

2 Lower to starting position.

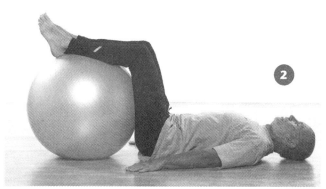

VARIATION: Place your arms across your chest and perform the movement.

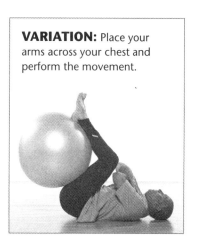

This advanced exercise requires good core stabilization. It engages your hamstrings and gluteal muscles.

STARTING POSITION: Lie on the floor on your back with your legs comfortably extended and lower legs resting on the exercise ball. Rest your arms alongside your body.

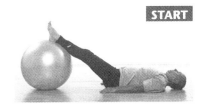

START

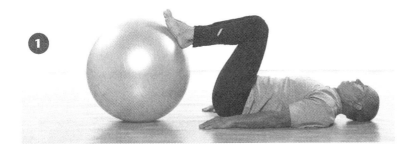

1 Press your heels into the ball while simultaneously rolling the ball toward your butt. Hold.

2 Extend your legs back to starting position and realign to neutral position.

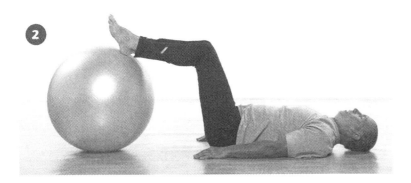

VARIATION: Perform the movement with your butt off the floor, but be careful to avoid getting hamstring cramps.

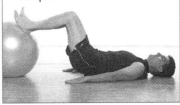

This exercise engages and strengthens the gluteal and low back muscles.

CAUTION: Be careful of hamstring cramps.

STARTING POSITION: Lie on the floor on your back with your lower legs extended and calves resting on the exercise ball. Locate neutral spine. Extend your arms along your sides.

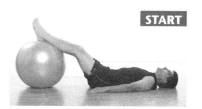

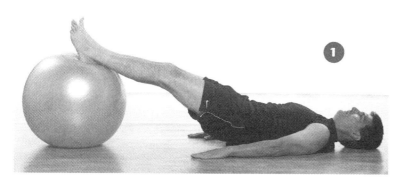

1 Maintaining neutral spine position, press the backs of the legs into the ball, elevating your butt off the floor. Make sure there are no spikes or dips in your posture. Hold.

2 Lower to starting position and relocate neutral spine position before performing the next rep.

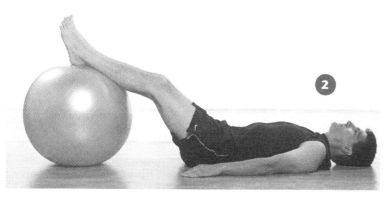

This exercise strengthens the spinal extensor muscle group, gluteus maximus, and shoulders. It also teaches body awareness.

CAUTION: Be alert to any increase in low back discomfort.

STARTING POSITION: Rest your chest or belly on the ball and place your hands on the floor for support. Extend your legs behind you and place your toes on the floor. Stabilize your low back by engaging your abdominal and low back muscles.

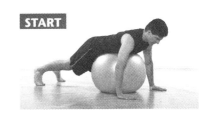
START

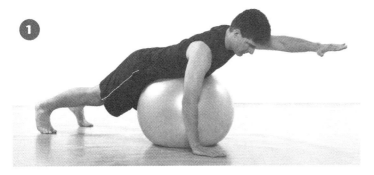
1

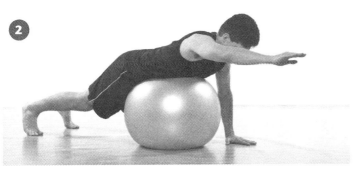
2

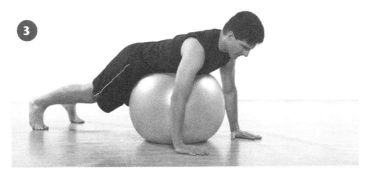
3

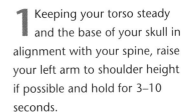

1 Keeping your torso steady and the base of your skull in alignment with your spine, raise your left arm to shoulder height if possible and hold for 3–10 seconds.

2 Lower your arm to the floor, then raise your other arm.

3 Lower your arm to the floor.

MODIFICATION: If your shoulders are inflexible, you can turn your thumbs up and move your arms up slightly to the side.

VARIATION: For an extra challenge, try raising both arms simultaneously.

This exercise strengthens the spinal extensor muscle group and gluteal region. It also teaches body awareness.

CAUTION: Be alert to any increase in low back discomfort.

STARTING POSITION: Rest your chest on the ball and place your hands on the floor for support. Extend your legs behind you and place your toes on the floor. Stabilize your low back by engaging your abdominal muscles.

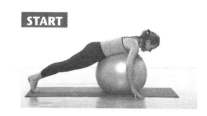

START

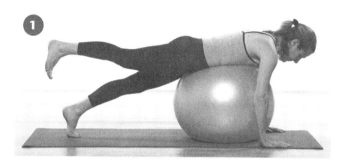

1 Keeping your torso steady and the base of your skull in alignment with your spine, raise your right leg no higher than hip height and hold for 3–10 seconds.

2 Lower your foot to the floor.

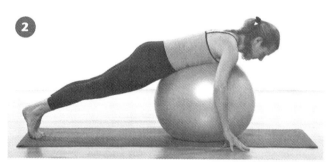

3 Raise your left leg no higher than hip height and hold for 3–10 seconds.

Lower your foot to the floor.

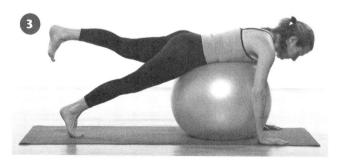

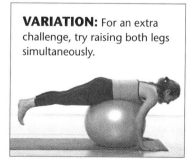

VARIATION: For an extra challenge, try raising both legs simultaneously.

This exercise strengthens the spinal extensor muscle group, gluteus maximus, and shoulders. It also teaches body awareness.

STARTING POSITION: Rest your chest on the ball and place your hands on the floor for support. Extend your legs behind you and place your toes on the floor. Stabilize your low back by engaging your abdominal muscles.

START

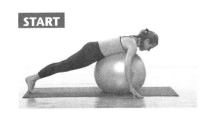

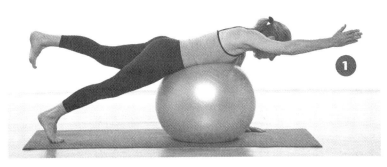

1 Keeping your torso steady and the base of your skull in alignment with your spine, raise your right arm and left leg to a comfortable height.

2 Lower to starting position.

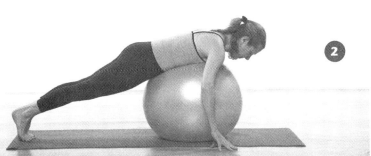

3 Raise your left arm and right leg to a comfortable height.

Lower to starting position.

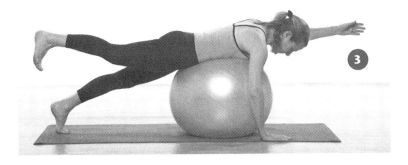

This exercise strengthens the lumbar extensor and gluteal muscle groups.

CAUTION: Do not overdo this exercise as you may trigger a low back muscle spasm. If you notice any discomfort, cease this move.

STARTING POSITION: Rest your chest or belly on the ball. Extend your legs behind you and place your toes on the floor. Stabilize your low back by engaging your abdominal muscles. Place your hands behind your head.

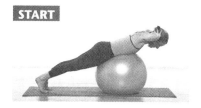

START

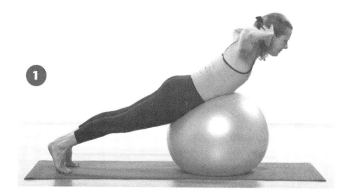

1 Slowly contract your low back muscles and squeeze your gluteal muscles to gently lift your torso a few inches off the ball.

2 Lower yourself to the ball.

Once you've finished your reps, curl your body around the ball to relax your low back muscles.

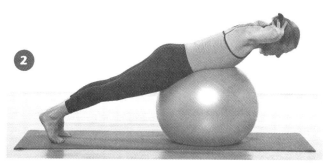

MODIFICATION: You can also do this with your hands on the floor, letting them lift as you raise off the ball.

ball series
ball plank

This is a very advanced exercise that simultaneously engages all the muscles of the core.

STARTING POSITION: Lie face-down on the ball with the ball under your thighs. Place your hands shoulder-width apart on the floor for support.

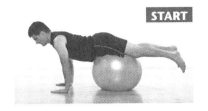

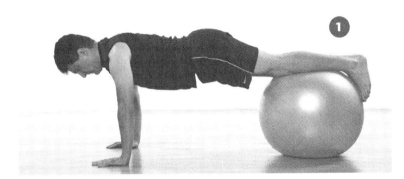

1 Slowly walk your hands forward, allowing the ball to roll down along your legs. Do not allow your back to arch or sag. The farther the ball goes down your legs, the more challenging the exercise becomes.

Slowly and cautiously return to starting position.

This super-advanced exercise simultaneously engages the muscles of the core along with the upper torso.

STARTING POSITION: Place the ball under your pelvic region and place your hands shoulder-width apart on the floor. Slowly walk your hands forward, allowing the ball to roll down to your shins. Do not allow your back to arch or sag.

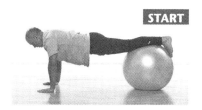

START

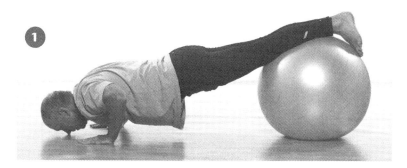

1 Keeping your back straight, bend your elbow to lower your chest toward the floor. Only go as far as you can while still maintaining proper alignment.

2 Slowly and cautiously press up to starting position.

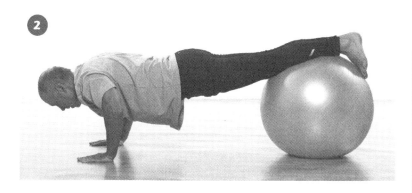

VARIATION: For an extra challenge, perform the push-up by placing your hands in a diamond shape or spreading your hands wide. You can also place your feet on the floor and your hands on the ball.

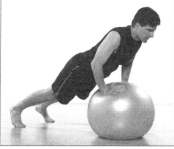

This exercise fosters better posture and leg strength.

STARTING POSITION: Place the ball between your low back and the wall.

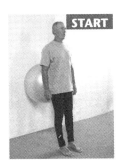

START

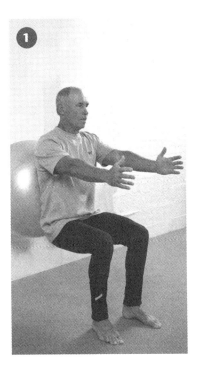

1

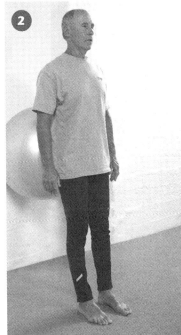

2

1 Bend your knees and hips and, if possible, lower yourself until your thighs are parallel to the floor. You may raise your arms for balance if necessary. Hold momentarily.

2 Slowly return to upright position.

This exercise engages many of the core muscles in a dynamic motion. Any object, including a basketball, tennis ball, or even a book, will suffice.

CAUTION: If rotation bothers your back, avoid this exercise.

STARTING POSITION: Stand back to back with your partner with one partner holding an object.

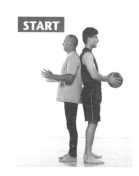

START

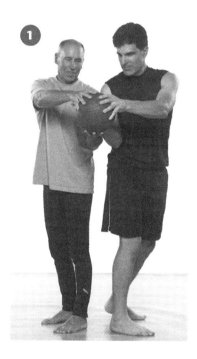

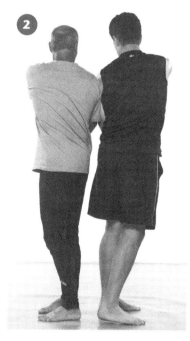

1 The partner with the object twists to the side and passes it to the other partner, who twists to receive the object. The partners pass the object to the same side several times.

2 The partners then repeat the twists to the opposite direction several times.

This exercise engages the complete kinetic chain of the core and works on spinal stabilization, so don't sacrifice form. Maintain proper alignment at all times. Once one partner either sags or arches his/her back, stop the exercise.

STARTING POSITION: Both partners assume a plank position on their hands and toes, about an arm's distance from each other.

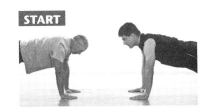

START

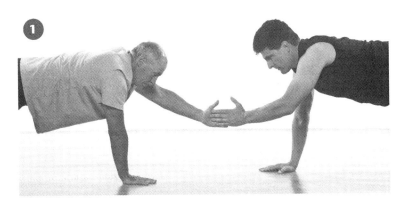

1 While in the plank position, one partner raises his/her right arm while the other partner raises his/her left arm so that you can clap hands.

2 After finishing reps on one side, swap positions so that you're now clapping with the other hand.

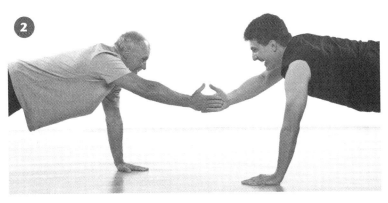

STARTING POSITION: Stand with proper posture.

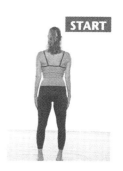

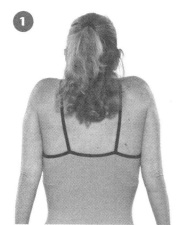

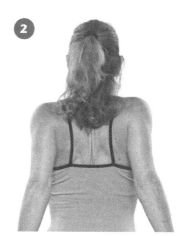

1 Inhaling deeply through your nose, slowly shrug your shoulders.

2 Now pull your shoulders back and squeeze the shoulder blades together and down.

3 Exhaling through your lips, drop your shoulders and return to starting position.

Repeat as desired.

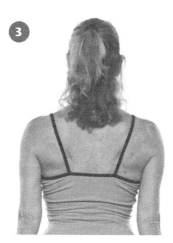

STARTING POSITION: Stand with proper posture. Position your hands in front of your body and interlace your fingers.

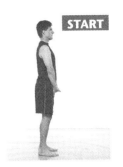

START

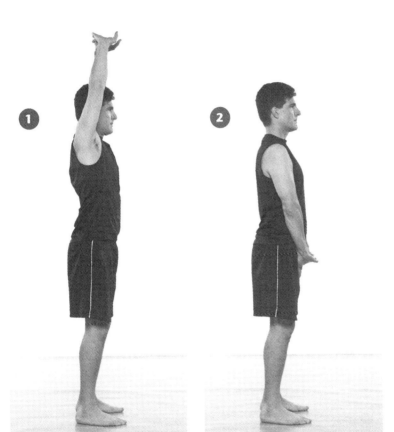

1 Inhale deeply through your nose and slowly raise both arms in front of you to a comfortable height. Hold for 1–2 seconds.

2 Slowly lower your arms to starting position.

Repeat as desired.

STARTING POSITION: Stand with proper posture and place your hands on your shoulders.

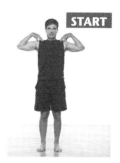

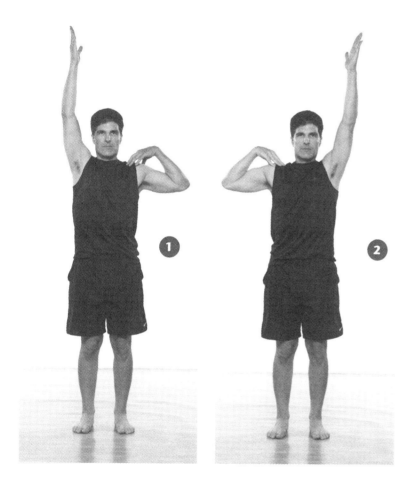

1 Reach your right hand as high as is comfortable.

2 Place your right hand back on your shoulder. Now reach up with your left hand.

Repeat as desired.

108 pec stretch

STARTING POSITION: Stand with proper posture. Place your hands behind your head.

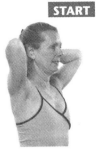

1 Gently move your elbows back and try to bring your shoulder blades together. Focus on opening up the chest and tightening the upper back muscles. Only go as far back as is comfortable and hold for a moment.

Repeat as desired.

1

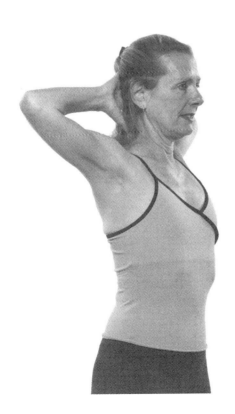

You can also use a bar instead of a strap.

STARTING POSITION: Stand with proper posture. Hold the ends of a strap in each hand behind your rear end.

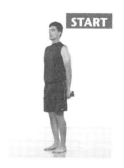

START

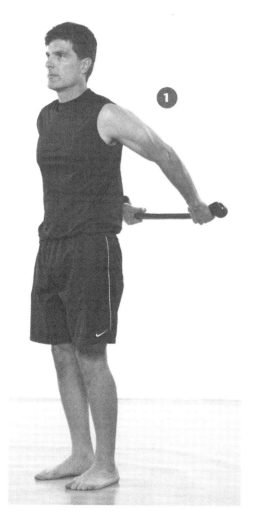

1 Attempt to straighten your arms behind you. Focus on squeezing your shoulder blades together. Avoid arching your back. Hold this position for as long as is comfortable.

ADVANCED: Instead of using a strap, interlock your hands behind your back.

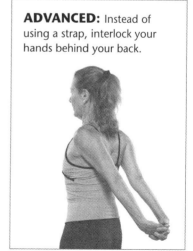

stretches
side bend

CAUTION: Be careful if you have low back pain.

STARTING POSITION: Stand with proper posture.

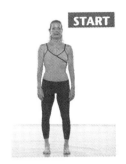
START

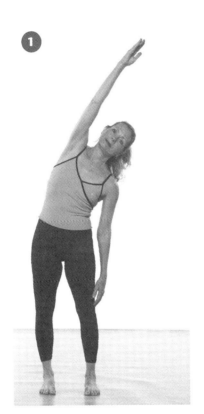
1

1 Raise your right arm over your head to a comfortable height. Inhale deeply through your nose then exhale through your lips and slowly and carefully lean to the left. Once you've leaned over enough to feel a gentle stretch along the right side of your body, hold this position for a comfortable moment.

Switch sides.

MODIFICATIONS: If your shoulder is stiff, place your hand on top of your head.

If raising your arm at all is very painful, just leave your arm alongside your body.

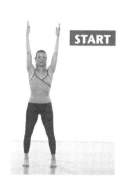
START

CAUTION: *If you have poor balance or low back problems, avoid this move.*

STARTING POSITION: Stand with proper posture. Raise your hands overhead with your arms as straight as feels comfortable. Inhale deeply through your nose.

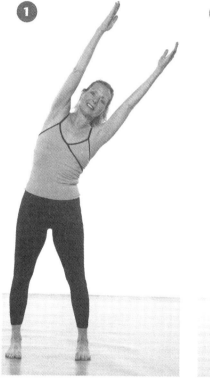

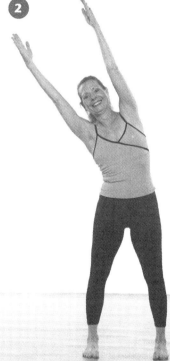

1 While exhaling through your lips, slowly lean to your left. Hold the position for a comfortable moment, feeling the stretch along the right side of your body.

2 Now inhale fully and deeply through your nose, then lean to your right. Hold this position for a comfortable moment.

ADVANCED: Try pressing your hands together as you do the side bends.

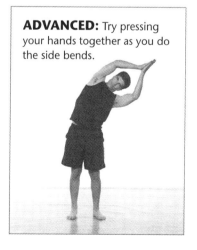

CAUTION: Avoid this exercise if you have poor balance. STOP if you notice undue compression in your knee or experience any low back discomfort. If you feel a cramp coming on, do a hamstring stretch.

THE STRETCH: Stand with proper posture. Bring your right heel toward your bottom and hold your ankle with your right hand. Keep both knees as close together as possible. Gently pull your heel closer to your bottom. Hold this stretch for a comfortable moment.

Switch sides.

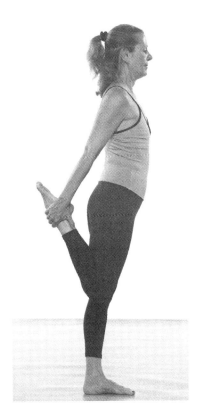

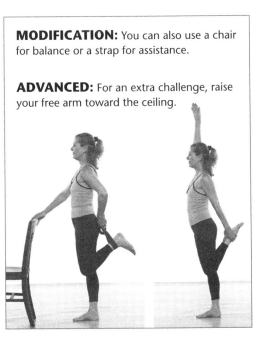

MODIFICATION: You can also use a chair for balance or a strap for assistance.

ADVANCED: For an extra challenge, raise your free arm toward the ceiling.

CAUTION: *Be careful if you have low back problems.*

You can also try this stretch while standing with proper posture.

STARTING POSITION: Sit with proper posture in a stable chair. Cross your arms in front of your chest and inhale slowly and deeply through your nose.

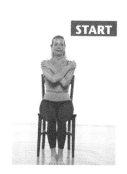

1 While exhaling through your lips, slowly twist to your left. Hold the position for a comfortable moment and feel the stretch in your torso.

2 Inhale and return to starting position before exhaling and twisting to your right. Hold the position for a comfortable moment and feel the stretch in your torso.

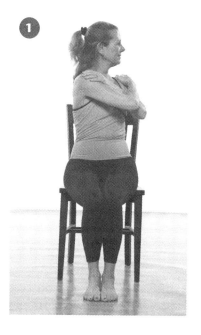

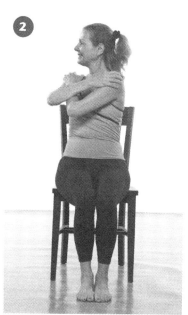

CAUTION: Avoid this move if you have knee problems.

THE STRETCH: Sit on a mat with both legs extended straight out in front of you. Keep your torso as tall as possible. Place your right foot against your left knee. Loop a strap around the sole of your left foot and hold on to the ends of the strap. Inhale deeply through your nose. While keeping your head and torso tall, exhale and pull yourself forward until you feel a comfortable stretch in the backs of your legs. Hold this stretch for a comfortable moment, focusing on the sensation of the stretch, not on going as far as possible. The goal is to hold the stretch for 60 seconds. Exhale through your lips and relax.

Switch sides.

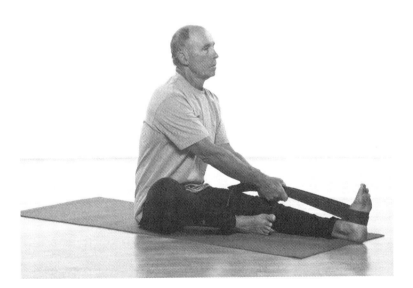

CAUTION: *If you have low back problems, avoid this move.*

STARTING POSITION: Lie on a mat with your knees bent and your feet flat on the floor. Place your arms straight out to your sides in a "T" position.

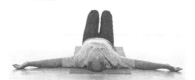

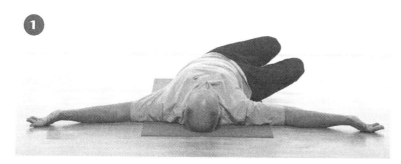

1 While inhaling through your nose, allow your knees to drop gently to the right without discomfort. Exhale and hold this position for a comfortable moment.

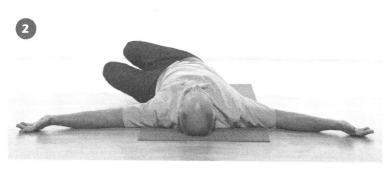

2 Inhale and bring your knees back to center, then gently drop them to your left. Exhale and hold this position for a comfortable moment.

CAUTION: Be careful if you have low back problems.

STARTING POSITION: Lie on a mat with your knees bent and your feet flat on the floor.

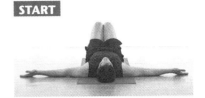
START

1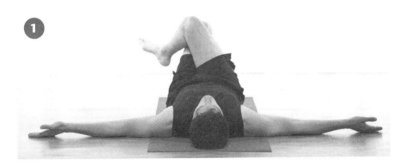

2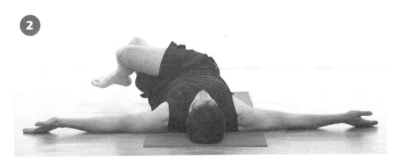

1 While focusing on your breathing, place your right knee on top of your left knee.

2 Slowly allow your right knee to gently fall toward the left side. Stop when you feel tightness. Hold this position for a comfortable moment. The stretch should be felt near the rear pocket area of the right leg. Focus on the stretch, not on how close you can bring the knees to the floor.

Switch sides.

single knee to chest

THE STRETCH: Lie on a mat and, if needed, place a pillow under your head. Extend both legs along the floor. Loop a strap behind the back of your right leg and hold an end of the strap in each hand. Gently pull the straps to bring the knee toward your chest. Hold this stretch for a comfortable moment.

Release the knee and switch sides.

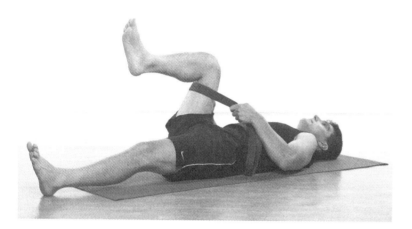

MODIFICATION: This can also be done with one knee bent with the foot on the floor.

VARIATION: This can also be done using just the hands to bring in the knee.

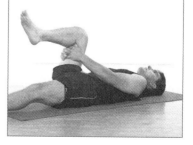

stretches
double knee to chest

THE STRETCH: Lie on a mat and, if needed, place a pillow under your head. Bend your knees, loop a strap behind the backs of both legs, and hold an end of the strap in each hand. Gently pull the straps to bring your knees to your chest. Hold this position for a comfortable moment, feeling the stretch in your bottom and low back.

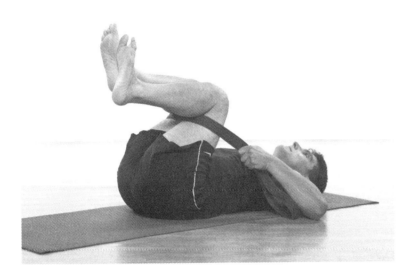

VARIATION: Use just your hands to draw in your knees.

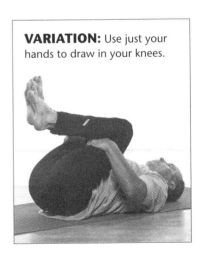

The piriformis muscle is a deep-lying muscle in the gluteal region, through which the sciatic nerve passes. When the piriformis is too tight, it can cramp the sciatic nerve, causing the symptoms of sciatica.

THE STRETCH: Lie on a mat and cross your right knee on top of your left knee. Loop a strap around both legs and pull your knees in toward your chest. Stop when tension occurs. Hold this position for a comfortable moment, focusing on the sensation of the stretch.

Switch sides.

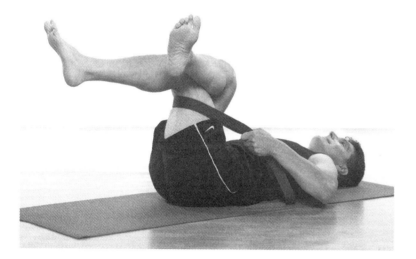

VARIATION: Use only your hands to pull your knees in.

STARTING POSITION: Lie on a mat and slowly bring both knees toward your chest. Gently reach around both legs and allow your shoulders to lift off the mat.

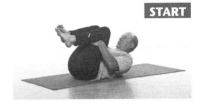

START

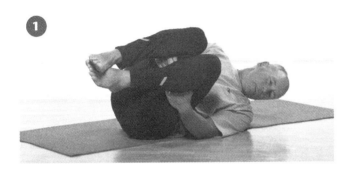

1

1–2 While inhaling deeply through your nose and exhaling through your lips, slowly rock left and right, enjoying the relaxing feeling.

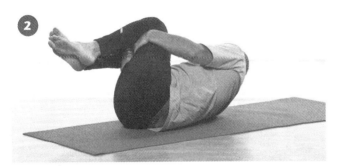

2

STARTING POSITION: Assume the tabletop position.

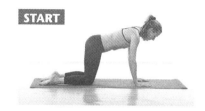

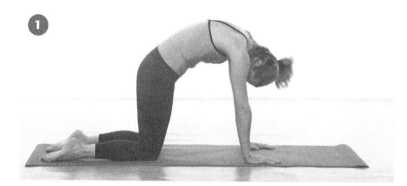

1 Draw your belly button in, causing your back to round. Inhale deeply.

2 Now exhale and slowly relax your body to the starting position.

Repeat as desired.

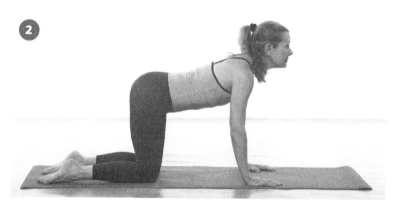

index

other books by karl knopf

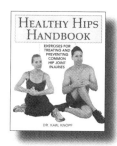

Healthy Hips Handbook
$14.95
Healthy Hips Handbook is designed to help prevent hip problems for some and, for those with existing hip problems, provide post-rehabilitation exercises.

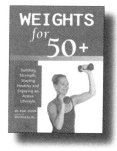

Weights for 50+
$14.95
Weight training is one of the most effective ways to get healthy and fight the physical signs of aging. *Weights for 50+* shows how easy it is for anyone to get started with weights.

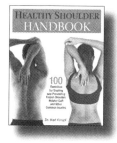

Healthy Shoulder Handbook
$15.95
Includes an overview of shoulder anatomy so anyone can use this friendly manual to strengthen an injured shoulder, identify the onset of a shoulder problem, or better understand injury prevention.

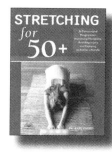

Stretching for 50+
$14.95
Based on the belief that individuals over 50 can do most of the same things as 20- and 30-year-olds, this book shows how to maintain and improve flexibility by incorporating stretching into one's life.

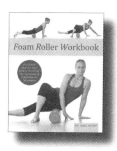

Foam Roller Workbook
$14.95
Details a comprehensive program for using the foam roller to recover from injury, reverse everyday pain, and stay healthy in the future.

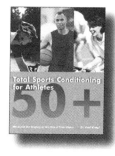

Total Sports Conditioning for Athletes 50+
$14.95
Provides sport-specific workouts that allow aging athletes to maintain the flexibility, strength, and speed needed to win.

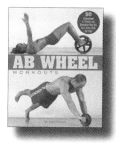

Ab Wheel Workouts
$14.95
With this book and an ab wheel, you'll rapidly develop a strong, lean physique, including sculpted abs, improved posture, toned upper body and greater athleticism.

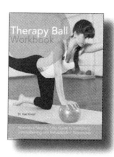

Therapy Ball Workbook
$14.95
Realize the full potential of massage balls for physical therapy, core strengthening, stability training, deep stretching, self massage and posture alignment.

To order these books call 800-377-2542 or 510-601-8301, fax 510-601-8307, e-mail ulysses@ulyssespress.com, or write to Ulysses Press, P.O. Box 3440, Berkeley, CA 94703. All retail orders are shipped free of charge. California residents must include sales tax. Allow two to three weeks for delivery.

acknowledgments

A special thanks goes to Lily Chou for sharing her insights and knowledge, which significantly improved the outcome of this book. Thanks also go out to the staff at Ulysses Press, whose support made this book possible. Additionally, a giant thank you to the models, Toni Silver and Jeff Rankin. Much appreciation also to the skilled photographic team at Rapt Productions. Lastly, a special thanks goes to my son Chris Knopf for his assistance with this book and to his mother Margaret for allowing me quiet time to work on this project when we could've been doing something fun.

about the author

KARL KNOPF, author of *Kettlebells for 50+, Foam Roller Workbook, Healthy Hips Handbook, Healthy Shoulder Handbook, Make the Pool Your Gym, Stretching for 50+, Weights for 50+,* and *Total Sports Conditioning for Athletes 50+,* has been involved with the health and fitness of the disabled and older adults for nearly 40 years. A consultant on numerous National Institutes of Health grants, Knopf has served as advisor to the PBS exercise series *Sit and Be Fit* and to the State of California on disabilities issues. He is a frequent speaker at conferences and has written several textbooks and articles. Knopf coordinates the Fitness Therapist Program at Foothill College in Los Altos Hills, California, and is the director of senior fitness at the International Sports Sciences Association (ISSA).